Handling Difficult Patients:

A Nurse Manager's Guide

RICHARD A. BRYAN, BSN, RN, CCM
LINDA CHILDERS

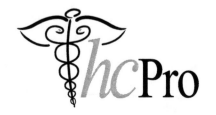

Richard A. Bryan, BSN, RN, CCM, Author
Linda Childers, Author
John Gettings, Associate Editor
Jean St. Pierre, Creative Director
Mike Mirabello, Senior Graphic Artist

Matthew Sharpe, Graphic Artist
Paul Singer, Layout Artist
Tom Philbrook, Cover Designer
Kathryn Levesque, Group Publisher
Suzanne Perney, Publisher

For more information, contact:
HCPro
P.O. Box 1168
Marblehead, MA 01945
Telephone: 800/650-6787 or 781/639-1872
Fax: 781/639-2982
E-mail: *customerservice@hcpro.com*

Visit HCPro at its World Wide Web sites:
www.hcmarketplace.com, *www.hcpro.com,* **and** *www.himinfo.com.*

Contents

Chapter 7: Improving Patient and Family Satisfaction in Specific Units 87

Chapter 8: Establishing Policies and Protocols 103

Chapter 9: Documenting the Difficult Patient Experience 135

Chapter 10: Leading Your Staff Toward Improved Service and Satisfaction 149

Chapter 11: Assessing Your Staff's Skills in Dealing with Difficult Patients and Families 161

Figures

About the Authors

Richard A. Bryan, BSN, RN, CCM

Richard A. Bryan, BSN, RN, CCM currently works as director of risk management and safety and security at Overlake Hospital Medical Center, Bellevue, WA. Richard has more than 10 years of experience in medical-legal consulting, case management, and risk management.

He has provided consultative services across the western United States to insurance companies, municipalities, governmental agencies, employers, attorneys, and health care facilities on a variety of medical-legal, case management, risk, and health related issues.

Spanning more than 20 years, Richard's health care background includes staff and management roles in medical-surgical, cardiac surgery, critical care, and emergency nursing in both civilian and military settings.

In addition to his duties at Overlake, Richard continues his active nursing practice at a rural hospital emergency department. He also serves as a commissioned officer in the United States Naval Reserve.

Linda Childers

Linda Childers has more than 15 years of experience working as a professional communicator. Five years ago, she founded her own company, Childers Communications, a Northern California-based communications firm.

Before founding her own company, Linda served as public information officer for Kaiser Permanente in one of their largest service areas, where she produced a number of publications for both Kaiser Permanente members and medical staff.

Linda writes on health care issues for a variety of hospitals, health plans, and other health care organizations. Her articles have been published in *NurseWeek, Minority Nurse, Healthplan, the San Jose Mercury News, Oakland Tribune, Contra Costa Times, ePregnancy, Fit Style, and the Farmers' Almanac.*

Linda began her writing career while still in high school, serving as a columnist for a major newspaper in the San Francisco Bay Area. In addition to being published in many local and regional publications, she has written many award-winning corporate publications. Linda holds a bachelor's degree in mass communication from California State University, Hayward.

Acknowledgements

My thanks are as follows:

To my mom, Marie Leonard Rosdahl, and dad, Rulon "Larry" Rosdahl for encouraging my love of reading and writing. I hope there are bookstores in heaven.

To my husband, Jeff, and son, Nikolas, for their unconditional love and support.

To my uncle, Robert Leonard, and cousin, Steve, for always caring

And to my friends, Stacey DeHart; Courtney Eisele; Denise Graham, RN; Patricia Griffith; Susan McGregor; Diane Roberti; and Kathy Sommese, RN. I couldn't ask for nicer friends or a better fan club!

And to Sierra and Truckee for sticking by me for the duration!

— Linda Childers

Introduction

Often in the medical profession, we fail to recognize that individuals seeking care bring with them the sum total of their experiences. These experiences are not limited to previous encounters with health care professionals and systems. They also include environmental, situational, and cultural aspects of their lives, as well as those of their family.

The complexities of living in our fast-moving society are only magnified when one seeks health care in any modern system. The rapidly evolving technology overwhelms even those of us who are familiar with it, so it becomes easy to see how laypeople may be affected. Add to this the need for treatment, be it associated with emergent or chronic conditions, and you have created a situation in which one additional stressor may tip someone over the edge.

This book is intended to provide insight and tools for both the new and seasoned health care manager as you attempt to meet the needs of a sicker and more complex patient population, including the elderly, immigrants/migrants, the uninsured, and the mentally ill and/or addicted patients. It is these groups of difficult patients, along with their families, that require increased resources, are at greater risk for negative encounters and outcomes, often have prolonged lengths of stay, and may lead to staff dissatisfaction.

As the frequency with which we encounter this patient population continues to grow, it is incumbent on all of us to work toward assessing the magnitude of the problem and developing methods by which we prevent problems from occurring while rapidly addressing those that do. It is critical that we implement changes that will enhance our ability to deliver quality, cost-effective care. It is our hope that the information contained within the book will prove useful in your quest to deal effectively with the difficult patient.

Chapter 1

DEFINING DIFFICULT
PATIENTS

CHAPTER 1

Defining Difficult Patients

Each day, hospitals and health care providers are presented with new challenges that compromise their ability to deliver care. These challenges include an ever-increasing regulatory environment; decreasing reimbursement; professional liability insurance premiums that have increased, in many instances by more than 250%; increasing labor, technology, supply, and pharmaceutical costs; and a growing shortage of qualified professionals. Despite these challenges, there is an expectation, and rightfully so, for the provision of quality health care to our communities.

In addition to regulatory and environmental issues, health care providers are faced with having to meet the needs of a sicker and more complex patient population. This population includes:

1. The elderly
2. Immigrants/migrants
3. Individuals with chronic mental illness and/or substance abuse
4. The uninsured

These particular patient populations are not exclusive in their requirement for

- increased resources
- prolonged lengths of stay
- increased risk for negative encounters and outcomes, and
- potential for staff dissatisfaction

They do, however, represent a significant portion of the population of patients served in most communities.

The following discussion is a closer look at each of those groups.

The elderly

According to the 2000 National Hospital Discharge Survey, conducted by the Centers for Disease Control (CDC), the elderly (those age 65 and older) comprised 40% of hospital discharges in 2000 versus 20% in 1970. These numbers become more alarming when presented in the context that all other age groups showed moderate declines during that same period.

The elderly undergo hospital procedures at a rate nearly three times the number of the next closest group. Procedures in the elderly are more frequently invasive in nature, as opposed to a higher number of diagnostic procedures in the other age groups. The average length of stay for a patient 65 years of age or older follows the trend at 6 days versus an average of 4.4 days for the remaining age groups.

Of noninstitutionalized adults, ages 70 and older, more than 24% were unable to perform at least one of nine physical functions. These functions included walking a quarter mile; walking up 10 steps without resting; standing or being on their feet for about two hours; sitting for about two hours; stooping, crouching, or kneeling; reaching up over their head; reaching out as if to shake someone's hand; using their fingers to grasp or handle; and lifting or carrying something as heavy as 10 pounds.

This data highlights the realities of what we in health care must deal with on a daily basis. They reflect the patient population that enters our facilities each day. This population, currently numbering approximately 35 million, is expected to double over the next 30 years to 70 million, with the fasting growing segment being the age group 85 and older.

The previous statistical information leaves little doubt about why this particular population requires more of our resources and poses a significant risk for poor outcomes and decreased satisfaction. Just the number of encounters with the health care systems raises the odds of an adverse event occurring.

Add to that chronic disabilities, functional deficits, memory loss, and depression, and the risk rapidly climbs.

Areas of particular risk in the elderly include:

1. Falls

2. Medication errors

3. Incorrect patient identification, leading to wrong procedures

4. Dehydration and skin breakdown

5. Increased confusion, leading to wandering or elopement

Each of these risks has potentially devastating consequences, and prevention efforts frequently require the commitment of extra resources.

Immigrant/migrant population

Although many geographic areas are experiencing substantial rates of growth in both legal and illegal immigrants, Health Status Indicators indicate that disparities in health care for most groups decreased. Areas that actually increased included work-related injury death rates, motor vehicle crash death rates, and suicide death rates. These types of occurrences remain troubling, and from a resource utilization standpoint, often represent episodes in which emergent treatment and trauma care was required. These types of episodes often create the need for critical care and may ultimately become end-of-life/withdrawal of life support scenarios.

Beliefs and opinions regarding end-of-life decision-making vary with regard to social and cultural groups. This variety may include appropriateness regarding the discussion of and planning for death, informing patients that they are dying, and the roles of individuals, family members, and physicians relative to end-of-life discussions.

Lack of cultural competency often leads to misunderstandings between the family and hospital staff caring for the patient. This will ultimately impede care, delay decisions, and affect the physical health of the patient and the emotional well-being of the staff involved.

Other potential sources of disparate treatment of this category of patients include:

1. Differences in socioeconomic status
2. Differences in health behaviors, including seeking treatment and following treatment recommendations
3. Discrimination and stereotyping by health care workers
4. Language barriers
5. Lack of diversity of our own staff
6. Lack of multicultural knowledge and sensitivity of our staff
7. Ability to access and pay for health care

Although health care providers face many of these issues on a regular basis, one of the most significant issues in dealing with the immigrant/migrant patient population is overcoming language barriers to health care. Thirty-two million people in this country, 13.8% of the population, speak a language other than English when at home, according to U.S. Census figures. Many of these individuals seek health care in our institutions and require qualified interpreters to describe potentially complex medical problems and treatment plans.

Translation of a medical visit by an unqualified interpreter could lead to omissions, additions, substitutions, volunteered opinions, and errors in semantics that have the potential to seriously affect care.

Congress passed Title VI of the Civil Rights Act to ensure that federal money is not used to support discrimination on the basis of race or national origin in government activities, including the delivery of health care. The language of Title VI includes the following instructions:

> *"No person in the United States shall, on the ground of race, color, or national origin, be excluded from participation in, be denied the benefits of, or be subjected to discrimination under any program or activity receiving Federal financial assistance."*

Since the majority of hospitals and health care providers receive compensation in the form of Medicare, Medicaid, and Tricare reimbursement, they are subject to the rules as set forth in a variety of governmental regulations, including Title VI.

Although the law does not call out language per se, the courts have consistently found a close connection between national origin and language. The U.S. Department of Health and Human Services' Office for Civil Rights (OCR) has also consistently found that those receiving federal funds have an obligation under Title VI to communicate effectively with those individuals with limited English proficiency. The agency has consistently set forth that "where language barriers cause persons with limited English proficiency to be excluded from or be denied equal access to health or social services, recipients may be required to take steps to provide language assistance to such persons."

In support of their position, the OCR has set forth the following basic requirements:

1. Recipients of federal funds should have a written policy for linguistic access and should make sure that staff are aware of the policy.

2. Recipients of federal funds should have a procedure for offering translation services to limited English proficiency patients during all hours of operation.

3. Family and friends should be allowed to interpret only after a patient has been informed of the availability of the services of a qualified interpreter at no cost to the patient.

4. Minors should not be used to translate.

5. "Qualified" interpreters should have demonstrated bilingual proficiency and knowledge of medical terms and the ethics of medical interpreting.

6. The use of telephone translation should be limited to situations in which no bilingual staff person or qualified interpreter is available to provide services.

7. Important medical documents should be translated for the patient.

The financial implications of providing the level of services as set forth in the OCR's guidelines are significant. More than a few providers have chosen to opt out of caring for any patients for whom any government funds are used for reimbursement. Although appropriate for their individual practices, this often results in a shift of care to hospitals or larger organizations, for whom opting out is not an option.

The lack of effective translation services clearly raises the cost of care. Many non-English–speaking patients are reluctant to work with health care providers who are unable to communicate in their native tongue. This results in their avoiding care until their conditions become more acute and/or emergent in nature. This is further supported by researchers in the Access Project, who determined that patients who experienced language barriers were less satisfied with their care, less likely to maintain one source of care, less likely to keep follow-up appointments, and less likely to receive preventive care.

Aside from the medical-legal implications, it becomes increasingly clear why we must pay close attention to the growing population of immigrants/migrants. The potential for harm is significant. Our approach must be directed toward increased cultural awareness, while taking into consideration the demand on resources and the impact on any organizations ability to deliver safe, quality care.

The uninsured

More than 43 million Americans had no health insurance coverage in 2002, according to the most recent estimate from the U.S. Census Bureau. This is an increase of more than 2.5 million people over the previous year and the largest annual increase over more than a decade of monitoring this key indicator of Americans' health and health care.

Data from The Kaiser Commission on Medicaid and the Uninsured indicates that the ranks of the uninsured are made up of low-income Americans (those earning less than 200% of the federal poverty level, or, for a family of three, $ 26,580.00 in 1999 dollars). The poor and the near poor make up 65% of the uninsured population.

Contrary to what many may believe, 83% of the uninsured are in working families. Also noteworthy is that immigrant households make up 26.1% of the nations uninsured. A newly emerging class of what would be characterized as underinsured is the elderly population, of which more than 10% live below the poverty level. Although eligible for some coverage under Medicare, out-of-pocket expenditures for deductibles, co-pays, and pharmaceutical costs exceed their ability to pay. It is anticipated that the percentages will continue to increase as the population continues to age.

Lack of health insurance not only takes a toll on families' financial well-being, it also compromises their ability to access health care in a timely manner, it also impacts their financial well-being. The Kaiser Family Foundation National Survey on the Uninsured 2000 revealed that nearly half of uninsured adults and one-fourth of uninsured children have no regular source of health care. Lack of health care coverage, when combined with the fear of incurring high medical bills, was reported to have resulted in delays or omission in necessary care.

The immediate impact on the uninsured's ability and/or willingness to obtain care is clearly demonstrated in the literature and data currently available. There is no doubt that it worsens the nature and severity of illness when they ultimately do seek care. Much more insidious, however, is the overall impact on health care providers and organizations, who are often faced with providing services to individuals with no ability to pay.

With approximately 14% of the population being uninsured, hospitals and health care providers are faced with a mounting burden of bad debt. Even in those instances where patients have the intent to pay, the reality is that they are often unable to do so. Adding to that burden is the total cost of uncompensated care, which in the year 2001 reached $ 21.5 billion dollars. This included the uninsured and the underinsured, as well as Medicare and Medicaid patients.

Those of us who are faced with the realities of providing care to the under- or uninsured population understand that this burden, which is anticipated to increase, has a negative impact on our ability to provide care. The cost of this burden comes at the expense of other programs, new technologies, staffing, and infrastructure. In short, it impacts our ability to deliver quality care.

The chronically mentally ill and substance abusers

According to the National Institutes of Mental Health, the current prevalence estimate is that approximately 28% of the U.S. population is affected by mental disorders in a given year. Of that number, 5.4% have "serious mental illness" and 2.6% have "severe and persistent mental illness."

When assessing the impact of the mentally ill patient, one must also take into consideration the fact that 9% of total mental health direct costs can be attributed to outpatient prescription drugs. The impact on health care institutions of this fact is profound, in that the significant lack of resources in this population results in their inability to maintain a stable drug regimen, which in turn results in cycles of noncompliance and the need for acute mental health services, including inpatient stabilization.

The impact of the mentally ill on acute care hospitals is profound. As data indicates, a significant number of the mentally ill have limited or no resources to pay for care. The absence of resources results in an increased demand on emergency services in order to prevent harm. The very nature of emergency departments leaves them ill equipped to provide the type of treatment required by the chronically mentally ill. In fact, the very presence of the acutely mentally ill can often tax the available resources of the emergency department, as the staff and physician attempt to ensure the patient's safety and identify the appropriate resources necessary for a safe disposition.

When asked, many health care providers identify drug seekers as having the greatest impact on their organizations. Although drug seekers do place an increased demand on resources, their numbers are difficult to accurately quantify. What is known is that, according to a 1999 study by the National Institute on Drug Abuse, nearly 2% of the population age 12 or older (approximately 4 million people) used prescription drugs nonmedically in the previous month. Although all of these patients do not obtain these drugs from acute care facilities, the impact remains significant.

Of equal importance is the impact of overall drug abuse on hospitals and emergency departments. The Drug Abuse Warning Network (DAWN) produced data for the year 2000 related to emergency department visits associated with drug abuse. The survey incorporated data from 466 hospitals in 21 metropolitan areas throughout the United States, from 1999-2000, including the following:

- Alcohol-in-combination (with other drugs) was the most frequently mentioned drug at the time of Emergency Department (ED) admission, followed by cocaine, heroin/morphine, and marijuana.
- ED visits related to the club drug ecstasy increased 58%, from 2,850 to 4,511.
- ED visits involving heroin/morphine increased 15%, from 84,409 to 97,287.

Among drug-related ED visits in 2000, dependence and suicide were the most frequently cited motives for drug ingestion. Overdose was the most common reason given for contacting an ED. Add to these statistics the numbers of events that often result from impaired individuals, including motor-vehicle crashes and other traumatic injuries, as well as injuries associated with drug-related crimes.

It becomes evident that drug addiction and drug-seeking behaviors have a significant effect on health care. A significant portion of this population is not insured. They often require emergency treatment, and in some instances require complex and long-term medical and surgical interventions. This population is also known to be at a higher risk for communicable diseases, including hepatitis and human immunodeficiency virus (HIV).

With both the mentally ill and the addicted patient population, health care providers face financial and emotional challenges. The financial impact notwithstanding, there is also an affect on human capital. This patient population results in significant demand on staff time and emotional energy.

Identification of resources and the ultimate potential for failure of even the best laid plan due to relapse or lack of follow-through often creates the need for more work and a profound sense of frustration on the part of those involved.

Traditionally, this population's disorders result in a decreased likelihood that they will follow treatment regimens and long-term treatment plans, which typically means frequent relapses and hospitalizations. Staff members may find themselves working on the same difficult patients month after month. The patients in this population often have personality conflicts with staff that may emerge as confrontational communication styles, manipulation, dishonesty, and mistrust. In all of these instances, staff have to work past their personal biases and frustrations to ensure that appropriate treatment is provided.

Facing the challenge

In this chapter, I have reviewed information and data that we as managers and health care providers are forced to live with every day. It is the reality of our world, yet it is the piece we were least prepared for when we entered the profession.

Even today, many clinicians fail to recognize the peril we now face as an industry. It is only through early identification of your institution's vulnerable points that you will then be able to take steps to meet the needs of your community today, and, more importantly, be there for them in the future.

How do we prevent harm to those individuals who walk through our doors seeking care and our staff assigned to those individuals?

How do we appropriately assess and treat populations with known compliance issues as we attempt to allocate our limited resources?

How do we maximize our utilization of resources in the face of dwindling reimbursement?

What is cultural competency, and what does that mean to our organizations?

How do we rally the financial and emotional resources necessary to care for our mentally ill and addicted patient populations?

In subsequent chapters, we will address specific issues regarding these difficult patient groups and their families. There are tools and methods by which we can improve the delivery of care and, ultimately, patient outcomes and bottom lines as well.

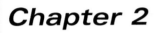

Chapter 2

DEALING WITH DIFFICULT FAMILIES

CHAPTER 2

Dealing with Difficult Families

Some are fearful, and some are angry because of a previous encounter with a health care professional. The reasons that patient families become "difficult" are as varied as the families themselves.

Nurses are often the primary contact with a patient's family. It is quite possible that a family who visits a family member in the hospital may never see the physician treating their loved one if their visits don't coincide with the times that a physician is conducting rounds.

Studies have shown that a majority of malpractice suits are brought not necessarily because of a bad outcome in treatment, but because patients and their families feel medical staff either lied to or stonewalled them. Many patients and their families seek legal representation because they believe the health professionals they dealt with showed no concern or warmth, wouldn't listen, wouldn't talk, or wouldn't answer questions.

Promoting open, honest communication with families

Creating an open, honest, and respectful communication environment with families is your first line of defense against difficult behavior and litigation. When this type of environment exists, families who feel they are being stonewalled or lied to are more likely to seek answers from you and your staff instead of an attorney.

Take a moment to analyze your environment. Think about what kind of relationship your organization has with patient families. Make sure everyone in your organization is doing all he or she can to effectively communicate and apply good service principles to patients' families.

There are some common situations and interactions within your organization that demonstrate your vulnerability to difficult patient/family litigation.

A poor office experience

Long waits, especially those without an apology or frequent check-ins, frustrate patients and families. This also may be an opportunity for an attorney to show a disorganized or hurried staff.

Make sure the communication climate is set from the moment a patient or family enters your facility. Does your receptionist make eye contact and say hello to everyone? When a patient or family member is called from the waiting area, does the nurse simply shout out a name and then turn around, expecting the family member to follow? Does your facility have a method for assuring no one patient or family member is kept waiting too long?

Family concerns met with lack of respect

Be aware of staff talking down or speaking in a judgmental way to patients or families. Do your nurses often interrupt patients or families? Do they appear to take their claims lightly? A difficult patient tends to remember these interactions for a long time.

Crucial information or developments are not delivered to the family

The physician scheduled to see the patient is replaced at the last minute by a colleague. This situation is not explained to the patient's family. A complication or error occurs during the exam. When the new physician speaks to the family, their first response is "Who are you?" This type of oversight will quickly transform your communication environment from one that is open and honest to one that is blanketed in mistrust.

Family inquiries met by vague nonanswers

Concerned loved ones seeking information about a patient can become difficult if their inquiries are met by vague responses.

Informed consent is mistaken for true understanding

A nervous patient may give his or her informed consent for a procedure but may not understand what the physician is communicating. The following day, the patient or loved one could call the office and ask for more details. The staff may not have time to walk the patient through all the information again. The patient or family member cannot get his or her questions answered and becomes angry when a complication occurs. This is an opportunity for a lawyer to show how the patient was denied important information.

Keeping your conversations with families constructive

Many nurse managers have found that an open and honest approach with a patient's family allows them to have a constructive conversation without either side feeling defensive.

Here are some tips for speaking with family members that become difficult:

Keep the conversation centered on the needs of the patient. Review the patient's current situation and the care plan with the family. If the family questions the care plan, ask for their input. "Are there any diagnostic tests or treatments you feel could help?" If they threaten to pursue a lawsuit, nurses can simply agree that is an option available to all families.

Ensure them that you are there to help, not take control. Families are often fueled by fear and feelings of helplessness and anger over the decline of their family member's health. By threatening to sue, patients and families are making an effort to regain a sense of control over a situation in which they feel powerless. By keeping the lines of communication open with families, updating them on new developments, showing empathy for their situation, and suggesting support groups or resources, many nurses have been successful in reducing the threat of litigation.

Empower them with knowledge. When an individual is diagnosed with a disease or admitted to the hospital, chances are that family members know very little about the condition and may fear the worst. Direct family members to your patient education department or wherever your organization provides resource materials. By directing them to valuable fact sheets and reference materials, you will help them gain knowledge about their family member's condition and potentially help them formulate specific questions to ask the doctor.

Help them realize they aren't alone. Having a family member hospitalized can be an incredibly isolating experience. Keep informed on support groups both within the hospital and in the community that are available to families as a resource. If possible, introduce them to "mentors," other families who are experiencing the same challenges.

When a family whose mother was just diagnosed with renal failure meets another family who is fighting the same battle, it can be an empowering experience as they share suggestions for caring for their loved ones and dealing with the day-to-day challenges of a chronic illness.

Make them part of the care process. When a family member is ill, families can feel helpless and out of control. It is important to keep them "in the loop." Nurse managers need to instruct nurses to suggest ways that families can offer assistance and feel like contributing members of the care team. Maybe they can read the morning newspaper to a family member, paint their fingernails, assist with feeding or bathing, or offer words of encouragement during physical therapy. Even little tasks can help make families feel they are doing something to support their loved one.

One long-term care facility created a communication book in the residents' rooms for encouraging communication and involvement between the staff and family. It was a way for the two parties that need to be involved in the patient's care to communicate social interactions—nothing in the book was related to care issues. Entries included:

- Your father played the piano at yesterday's holiday party. He really enjoyed it.
- Your mother is due for her hair appointment. Would you like to schedule it?

Strategies for providing quality family care

- Encourage nurses to take the lead by introducing themselves to a patient's family, providing an overview of the patient's condition, meds, and so on, and asking the family if they have any questions. The bedside nurse can address many routine care questions, but if the questions need to be addressed by a physician, request that nurses leave a message, stating the nature of the question and asking the physician to contact the family at the earliest convenience.

- If a family is anxious about a patient's condition, encourage nurses to reassure families that they will be called immediately if there are any changes in the patient's condition. If the patient's family prefers to call for updates, inform them of the best time to call to avoid shift changes, report times, and so on. In some cases you may want to appoint a spokesperson for the family to contact.

- Take a team approach to care. A family that has just learned a relative is dying may need more emotional care than a nurse has the time to give. Train nurses to ask families if there is anyone they can call to support the family in their time of need and also offer the services of the hospital chaplain or social worker.

- Do your nurses provide follow-up care to patients and their families? Hospitals that have reported an increase in patient satisfaction scores have implemented programs in which nurses provide follow-up phone calls in areas such as ambulatory surgery and obstetrics to check on patients and get their feedback. This is also a good time to answer patient questions regarding discharge instructions and medications.

- How does your staff handle complaints or concerns from families? In many facilities, nurses encourage families to take their concerns to a specific nurse administrator, since floor nurses have little time to deal with problems that may be systemic. Are nurses familiar with your protocols for handling concerns? Are concerns addressed within a reasonable amount of time?

How to respond to an angry complaint

Anger-fueled complaints are part of the territory for nurses. Susan Keane Baker, a motivational speaker in the health care field, offers these steps for handling angry complaints from patients and their families.

Try role-playing these strategies with your nursing staff.

- Move the patient or family member to a quiet area. In a low, calm voice, nurses should say, "Let's step over here to talk. That way we won't be interrupted." The angry patient or family member with an audience will be less likely to accept the nurse's point of view.

- Let the patient or family member speak his or her mind without interruption. Otherwise, the nurse may fix the problem, but not fix the relationship. By interrupting, nurses may inadvertently encourage the person to embellish and repeat his or her story to others. Patients and their families have a need to feel they are being heard and taken seriously.

- Avoid rationalizing. There are usually a few oft-repeated rationalizations that come immediately to mind when a patient or family member has a complaint. Put yourself in the patient's shoes for just a moment and consider whether your rationalization is an explanation or an excuse.

- Respectfully use the name of the patient or family member in your reply. When a person is very angry, using his or her name in a respectful way can ease the situation. Using the person's name in a condescending way will likely spark anger.

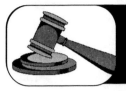

CASE STUDY: CALIFORNIA HOSPITAL INITIATES MONTHLY SUPPORT GROUP

Administrators at a long-term care facility in California joined forces with patient families to form a monthly support group.

Each meeting featured speakers who gave a presentation on a topic of interest to families. Since many of the patients had cognitive impairment, a representative from the local Alzheimer's administration offered families tips on how to effectively communicate with a loved one who has dementia.

A local pharmacist answered questions on frequently prescribed medications. Each meeting also included ample time for families to ask questions of the administrator, and for staff to report new information.

Families in the group formed a "phone tree" by which they could call upon each other to check on their loved ones while they were on vacation.

The support group gave families a chance to come together regularly with other caregivers for support and encouragement, and to increase their knowledge of the facility and various issues surrounding long-term care. Administrators found that the meetings improved communication with families and increased patient satisfaction.

Group appointments may offer solutions and support

Many medical facilities have started to offer group appointments to patients with chronic illnesses and their family members. These extended medical appointments are a wonderful way to bring together patients with the same questions and concerns and give them a chance to meet other patients and spend quality time with a physician and nurse educator.

Before establishing this service, however, the organization should check with counsel to ensure that the payment for these services will not put them in violation of anti-kickback statues. Unless these services are charged back to the physician or the physician is an employee of the facility, group appointments could be a violation.

As a nurse manager, consider having your nursing staff join forces with physicians to offer group appointments. Families are invited to attend group appointments and can obtain information that will assist them in their roles as caregivers.

Nurses can assist at group appointments by taking patients' vital signs and also helping the physician with the educational presentation.

Group appointments are scheduled at regular times and usually last approximately two hours. They offer a supportive give-and-take environment for patients and their families, allowing them to ask questions about their illness or treatment. Patients and their families learn from each other and benefit from the group experience.

These appointments are most beneficial for patients who

- have a chronic condition such as asthma, arthritis, hypertension, diabetes, depression, or renal failure
- require routine follow-up appointments such as during a pregnancy
- typically require more time with their physician
- come for frequent return visits
- have extensive emotional, informational, or psychosocial needs

Promoting family-centered care

Many hospitals have begun implementing "family-centered care," a practice that places the patient's family at the forefront of treatment.

This approach encourages health care providers and families to work together to meet the individual needs of each patient. By providing information and insights, families help nurses improve care. This team approach embraces respect for family, informed choices, information sharing, emotional support, collaboration, and empowerment.

In family-centered environments, there are comfortable accommodations so that a family member can stay overnight in a patient's room. Families aren't considered visitors but rather essential caregivers and participants who affect the total healing of the patient.

Although the concept of family-centered care originally started with pediatric facilities, the principles have translated well to adult care settings. By providing family-centered care, caregivers are discovering improved health outcomes for patients, increased job satisfaction for health care providers, and continuity of care for patients after they have been discharged from the hospital.

As part of the family-centered care concept, family members are connected with others dealing with similar health issues for emotional, spiritual, and practical support. Parents with a child being treated for cystic fibrosis might be connected with "parent peers" who can recall how they handled their own child's hospitalization and address the same concerns and challenges they faced.

Addressing family stress that may lead to difficult behavior

A hospitalization affects not only the patient but also family members and friends who often experience stress and uncertainty, which can manifest itself in difficult behavior when a loved one is admitted to the hospital. Once nurses understand what is causing the family stress, they are in a better position to offer help.

Concerns about information
Families are concerned about what is happening to their loved one in the hospital and how much information they will get. Families feel the helplessness of losing control of the patient's care and the frustration of not being able to ease a loved one's fear or pain.

Anxiety about care and finances after discharge
Families and friends worry that they may not be able to care for their loved one after discharge or that

they might not be able to pay for necessary care if a loved one needs to go to a long-term care facility. This dilemma is especially painful when family members live far away from the patient and have to make arrangements for care.

If you are concerned about the stress a family is experiencing and fear it may lead to a confrontation, here are some suggested interventions:

- Ask if they would like to speak to the hospital chaplain, social worker, or your patient relations representative.

- Increase the frequency of your updates on the patient's condition and offer to explain any medical equipment being used and its purpose.

- If your hospital utilizes "patient pathways" that outline the commonly expected daily plan of care for different medical conditions, offer to share this with the family.

- Chances are they had several questions for the physician but then forgot what to ask when the he or she was conducting rounds. Encourage the family to write down important questions they have for the physician.

- If family members have concerns regarding a patient's prognosis or part of the care plan and asks for a second opinion, explain that is their right and let them know they should feel comfortable making the right decisions.

Difficult families are a challenge for every health care organization. Poor communication with a patient's family can lead to staff dissatisfaction and an increased chance of a negative patient outcome. If you don't take the time examine your communication environment now, a lawyer may do it for you in the future. Families who feel as if they have been lied to or stonewalled by nurse often seek answers from an attorney, not you.

Handling difficult families effectively requires that you take closer look at the communication environment in which you work. You must recognize the stress these families are experiencing and use the strategies described in this chapter to relieve their anxiety. This means more than just listening with empathy. You have to make them aware of support channels, empower them with education, and make them a part of the care process—all in the name of good customer service.

Chapter 3

ASSESSING DIFFICULT PATIENTS

CHAPTER 3

Assessing Difficult Patients

The necessity for a comprehensive assessment and admission history should be apparent. It is the basis on which a plan of care is developed. Although time consuming, an accurate and complete admission assessment will increase the likelihood that we will be able to meet our obligation as a health care provider.

Many activities and associated risks will become more readily apparent. Assessments should include vulnerability points such as mental status, history of falls, functional status, and the presence of advanced directives.

After obtaining a comprehensive understanding of the patient's conditions and potential needs, case management and discharge planning should be initiated. Earlier it was noted that the continuum of care is best achieved through integration of planning and care throughout all of the patient environments.

The elderly patient remains one of the most at-risk populations within the hospital. Areas of concern include their risk for falls, the nutrition status, their ability to safely swallow or clear secretions, the condition of their skin, the numbers and types of medications they are on and their cognitive and mental status. In order to accurately care for these patients, there must be a comprehensive baseline assessment from which a plan of care can be derived.

Although most hospitals routinely incorporate skin and fall assessments into their admission process, there is a failure to act on the information that is collected. Development of a systematic approach to assessment, along with a plan for communication regarding conditions that may place a patient at risk, will serve the nursing staff well.

Early identification of at-risk patients allows for a proactive approach to ensuring that the patient remains safe throughout their hospitalization. The dividend is a reduction in injuries or adverse outcomes and the time and financial resources associated with dealing with those types of catastrophic events.

Cognitive assessment challenges

Although a lot of assessment functions are done well, the challenge for acute care settings is developing a process for more in-depth assessments, especially those that deal with cognitive function.

Acute care hospitals are still struggling with how to integrate the cognitive function into day to day procedure. Ideally there would be a consistent and effective approach for determining such things like whether this person is forgetful, a wonderer, an elopement risk, and so on. Long-term care facilities are doing a fairly good job at this, but at the same time, patients' cognitive challenges are usually more obvious at that point.

To better determine a patient's competency, clinical social workers at Overlake Hospital Medical Center use the assessment tool found in Figure 3.1. This Mini Mental State Exam is a more in-depth assessment and is used to assess things like the patient's future ability to make decisions for him or herself, get home, or determine whether guardian needs to be appointed.

Figure 3.1	**Mini Mental State Exam**

MINI - MENTAL STATE EXAM with Item-Response Calculation
standard version - Folstein, Folstein, McHugh, 1975
(to be completed by a trained clinician)

PATIENT NAME: _____

DATE:_____   TIME:_____

ENTER BIRTH DATE: _____ *(mmddyyyy)*

Sex: Male   Female   Enter education (years) _____

Race: Caucasian   Black   Hispanic   Asian   Other

Orientation Questions: Ask the following questions:

right   wrong

— — 1. What is today's date?

— — 2. What is the month?

— — 3. What is the year?

— — 4. What day of the week is today?

— — 5. What season is it?   DATE:_____

— — 6. What is the name of this clinic (place)?

— — 7. What floor are we on?

— — 8. What city are we in?

— — 9. What county are we in?

— — 10. What state are we in?   PLACE:_____

Early assessment of the mental status of patients may help you more effectively manage care for these patients and potentially prevent one from becoming difficult. Here are some common disorders and simple things for staff members to watch out for when these patients present in your facility:

- A patient who is depressed may have no appetite, mention a loss of interest in doing pleasurable things, withdraw from others, and have frequent sleep interruptions.

- A patient who may have a borderline personality disorder may exhibit manipulative behavior, pitting one staff member against another; direct their care the way they want it to go; and feel as if they are always right, and the staff is always wrong.

- A patient who is bipolar may show signs and symptoms of depression, coupled with instances of boundless energy; their ability to focus will be intermittent.

Signs of dementia

Dementia is very prevalent among the elderly but is often overlooked even by skilled clinicians. Clues to the presence of dementia may be subtle and nonspecific. The Alzheimer's Association and the National Chronic Care Consortium developed the following list of patient behavior triggers for clinical staff.

Individuals with undiagnosed dementia may exhibit behaviors or symptoms that offer a clue to the presence of dementia and can be observed by physicians, nurses, and other clinical staff. The need for early dementia recognition techniques is going to play a significant role in the care your organization delivers in the future. As discussed in Chapter 1, the number of patients with cognitive impairment that are seen in emergency rooms and hospitals is growing and will continue to grow in the foreseeable future.

Here are some examples of symptoms that may signal dementia:

The patient

- is a "poor historian" or "seems odd"
- is inattentive to appearance, inappropriately dressed or dirty
- fails to appear for scheduled appointments or comes at the wrong time or on the wrong day
- repeatedly and apparently unintentionally fails to follow instructions (e.g., changing medications)
- has unexpected weight loss, "failure to thrive," or vague symptoms (e.g., weakness or dizziness)
- seems unable to adapt or experiences functional difficulties under stress (e.g., the hospitalization, death, or illness of a spouse)
- defers to a caregiver—a family member answers questions directed to the patient

It may be helpful to follow up on areas of concern by asking the patient or family members relevant questions.

Family questionnaire to determine dementia

The Alzheimer's Association and the Chronic Care Consortium also developed the following family questionnaire to help clinicians identify patients with memory problems that might otherwise go unnoticed. It consists of five simple questions. A family member or friend of the patient can complete the questionnaire in less than a minute.

Use of the family questionnaire is encouraged for all patients who meet all of the following criteria:

- If the patient has no prior diagnosis of dementia
- If the patient is 65 or older
- If the patient comes to the clinic in the company of a family member or friend
- If the questionnaire has not been completed in the past year

How to use the Family Questionnaire

First, determine if a family member or friend has come in with the patient.

While you are checking vital signs and collecting other screening information, tell the patient you have a brief questionnaire for his or her family member or friend that will help medical staff determine if the patient has trouble remembering or thinking clearly. Explain that these symptoms may not come to the attention of medical professionals and that recognizing symptoms will allow clinicians to take better care of the patient. Be sure the patient consents; then present the questionnaire to the family member or friend.

Use the information on the questionnaire listed below when you explain it to the family member. Ask the family member to turn the questionnaire to you once it is completed. Score the questionnaire accordingly and attach it to the patient's chart.

Figure 3.2 **Family Questionnaire**

We are trying to improve the care of older adults. Some older adults develop problems with memory or the ability to think clearly. When this occurs, it may not come to the attention of the physician.

Family members or friends of an older person may be aware of problems that should prompt further evaluation by the physician. Please answer the following questions. This information will help us to better care for your family member.

In your opinion does _____ have problems with any of the following:
(Please circle the appropriate answer. Not at all, Mild (a little), or Severe (a lot).)

1. Repeating or asking the same thing over and over?	Not at all	Mild	Severe
2. Remembering appointments, family occasions and holidays?	Not at all	Mild	Severe
3. Writing checks, paying bills, balancing the checkbook?	Not at all	Mild	Severe
4. Deciding what groceries or clothes to buy?	Not at all	Mild	Severe
5. Taking medications according to instructions?	Not at all	Mild	Severe

Relationship to patient _____
(spouse, son, daughter, brother, sister, grandchild, friend, etc.)

Scoring:
Not at all = 0
Mild (a little) = 1
Severe (a lot) = 2   Total score _____

Score interpretation:
7-10, probable cognitive impairment
3-6, possible cognitive impairment
A score of 3 or more should prompt the consideration of a more detailed evaluation.

Signs of depression

The challenge with using any of these cognitive assessment tools is finding ways to work these into day-to-day procedure. To this end, the assessment tool found on p. 36 (Figure 3.3) was designed to help nurses and other clinicians screen patients for depression.

Depression is one of the most common and undiagnosed problems in the elderly. Early screening for depression may help staff better handle a patient's complex care planning needs. The Alzheimer's Association and the National Chronic Care Consortium developed this screening tool.

Suspected substance abusers

A patient who presents to the emergency department (ED) with alcohol or another substance abuse problem, is not likely to discuss his or her addiction or abuse problems openly with you. During your assessment of the patient, he or she could be intoxicated, in acute withdrawal, or in no apparent distress at all.

The following tools in Figure 3.4 are very basic assessment forms that helps answer important questions about suspected substance abusers.

Typically, with substance abuse patients, it is important that you include the family and their observations, otherwise you are not going to get an accurate picture.

We will discuss the importance of having a policy for dealing with these patients in Chapter 8.

Figure 3.3 **Geriatric Depression Scale**

Depression is one of the most common and undiagnosed problems in the elderly. The Alzheimer's Association and the National Chronic Care Consortium offer the following assessment tool to help nurses and other clinicians screen for depression.

1.	Are you basically satisfied with your life?	Yes	No
2.	Have you dropped many of your activities and interests?	Yes	No
3.	Do you feel that your life is empty?	Yes	No
4.	Do you often get bored?	Yes	No
5.	Are you in good spirits most of the time?	Yes	No
6.	Are you afraid that something bad is going to happen to you?	Yes	No
7.	Do you feel happy most of the time?	Yes	No
8.	Do you often feel helpless?	Yes	No
9.	Do you prefer to stay at home rather than going out and doing new things?	Yes	No
10.	Do you feel you have more problems with memory than most?	Yes	No
11.	Do you think it's wonderful to be alive now?	Yes	No
12.	Do you feel pretty worthless the way you are now?	Yes	No
13.	Do you feel full of energy?	Yes	No
14.	Do you feel that your situation is hopeless?	Yes	No
15.	Do you think most people are better off than you are?	Yes	No

Score_____(number of depressed answers)

Depressed answers are: No on numbers 1, 5, 7, 11, 13
Yes on numbers 2, 3, 4, 6, 8, 9, 10, 12, 14, 15

1-4 – No cause for concern
5-9 – Strong probability of depression
10+ – Indicative of depression
5 or more – Depressed answers warrant further evaluation

Figure 3.4	**Substance Abuse Screening Tools**

Brief Screening: TWEAK Test

This screening instrument is to be administered as part of a general screening.

Do you drink alcoholic beverages? If you do, please take our "TWEAK Test."

T	**Tolerance:** How many drinks does it take to make you feel high? (Record number of drinks) *Score 2 points if she reports 3 or more drinks to feel the effects of alcohol.* **Score:**____	**No. of drinks** ____
W	**Worry:** Have close friends or relatives worried or complained about your drinking in the past year? *Score 2 points for a positive "yes".* **Score:**____	____Yes ____ No
E	**Eye-Opener:** Do you sometimes have a drink in the morning when you first get up? *Score 1 point for a positive "yes".* **Score:**____	____Yes ____ No
A	**Amnesia (Blackouts):** Has a friend or family member ever told you about things you said or did while you were drinking that you could not remember? *Score 1 point for a positive "yes".* **Score:**____	____Yes ____ No
K(C)	**Cut Down:** Do you sometimes feel the need to cut down on your drinking? *Score 1 point for a positive "yes".* **Score:**____	____Yes ____ No
	Total Score = _____ *A total score of 2 or more points indicates a likely drinking problem.*	

Source: Russel, Marcia, Martier, Susan S., Sokol, Rober J., Mudar, Pamela, Bottoms, Sidney, Jacobsen, Sandra & Jacobsen, Joseph (1994). Screening for Pregnancy Risk-Drinking. *Alcoholism: Clinical and Experimental Research*, 18 (5): 1156-1161.

| Figure 3.4 | ■■■■■ **Substance Abuse Screening Tools (cont.)** ■■■■■ |

Brief Screening: T-ACE

T-ACE is a measurement tool of four questions that are significant identifiers of risk drinking (i.e., alcohol intake sufficient to potentially damage the embryo/fetus).
The T-ACE is completed at intake. The T-ACE score has a range of 0-5. The value of each answer to the four questions is totalled to determine the final T-ACE score.
Note:
1 Drink
= 12 oz beer
= 12 oz cooler
= 5 oz wine
= 1 mixed drink (1.5 oz. hard liquor)
Binge (drinking) = consuming 5 or more alcoholic drinks on an occasion
A total score of 2 or greater indicates potential risk for the purposes of Pregnancy Outreach Program identification of prenatal risk.

1. How many drinks does it take to make you feel high? 1. less than or equal to 2 drinks 2. more than 2 drinks	**Tolerance**
2. Have people annoyed you by criticizing your drinking? 1. No 2. Yes	**Annoyance**
3. Have you felt you ought to cut down on your drinking? 1. No 2. Yes	**Cut Down**
4. Have you ever had a drink first thing in the morning to steady your nerves or to get rid of a hangover? 1. No 2. Yes	**Eye Opener**
Total Score = _____	

Source:

Sokol, Robert J., "Finding the Risk Drinker in Your Clinical Practice" in G. Robinson and R. Armstrong (eds), Alcohol and Child/Family Health: Proceedings of a Conference with Particular Reference to the Prevention of Alcohol-Related Birth Defects. Vancouver, BC., December, 1988.

Figure 3.4	**Substance Abuse Screening Tools (cont.)**

Alcohol and Drug Assessment Questionnaire

Caffeine

How much of each of the following substances do you consume in a day? (greater than 400 mg/day = potential prenatal risk)

Substance	Pre-pregnancy	At intake
Coffee: - Perc - Drip - Instant	Daily consumption in cups ___ cups x 110 mgs = _____ mgs ___ cups x 145 mgs = _____ mgs ___ cups x 75 mgs = _____ mgs	Daily consumption in cups ___ cups x 110 mgs = _____ mgs ___ cups x 145 mgs = _____ mgs ___ cups x 75 mgs = _____ mgs
Tea - Regular - Herbal	Daily consumption in cups ___ cups x 65 mgs = _____ mgs ___ cups x 0 mgs = __0__ mgs	Daily consumption in cups ___ cups x 65 mgs = _____ mgs ___ cups x 0 mgs = __0__ mgs
Cola	___ cans x 35 mgs = _____ mgs	___ cans x 35 mgs = _____ mgs

Smoking

When was the last time you smoked cigarettes, if ever?
___ Never smoked
___ Within the last 2 weeks
___ Within the last month
___ Within the last 3 months
___ Within the last 6 months
___ Within the last year
___ Over 1 year ago

Before you were pregnant, how many cigarettes, on average, did you smoke in a week? _____

How many cigarettes, on average, did you smoke last week? (at prenatal intake) _____

Alcohol

When was the last time you drank alcohol, if ever?
___ Never drank alcohol
___ Within the last 2 weeks
___ Within the last month
___ Within the last 3 months
___ Within the last 6 months
___ Within the last year
___ Over 1 year ago

Before you were pregnant, how many times (occasions) did you drink alcohol each week? ____;
each month? ____
On average, how many drinks did you have on an occasion? _____

Is there any history of misuse of alcohol by any of the following family members?
___ Biological mother
___ Biological father
___ Spouse/partner
___ Brother/sister
___ None apply

Have you had any treatment for alcohol use?
___ Yes: Where? _____
When? _____
___ No

What is your understanding of the possible effects that drinking alcohol may have during pregnancy? (Fetal Alcohol Syndrome)?

| Figure 3.4 | Substance Abuse Screening Tools (cont.) |

Drugs

When was the last time you used drugs, if ever?
___ Never used drugs
___ Within the last 2 weeks
___ Within the last month
___ Within the last 3 months
___ Within the last 6 months
___ Within the last year
___ Over 1 year ago

Before you were pregnant, how many times (occasions), on average, did you use drugs each week?
____ ; each month? ____

In the past week, how many times did you use drugs? ____ (at intake)

Have you had any treatment for drug use?
___ Yes: Where? _____
      When? _____
___ No

Drugs Used (check all that apply)

Drug	Within 2 weeks	Within 1 month	Within 6 months	Within 1 year	Over 1 year ago
Marijuana/THC					
Crack/Cocaine					
Cocaine (IV)					
LSD/Acid					
Heroin (IV)					
Heroin (other)					
Tylenol/Codeine (T 3's)					
Barbiturates and other tranquillizers					
Other tranquillizers					
Inhalants					
Other (specify): _____					

Charlotte Kasl,© 1991, *Many Roads, One Journey: Moving Beyond the 12 Steps.*

The following are signs and symptoms to look for to help you better identify these patients:

Needle marks—Substance abusers injecting drugs will typically present with needle marks. These marks can be on any part of the body but are typically in the arms. Also be aware of patients who have abscesses or infections as a result of using dirty needles.

Erratic behavior—When you entered the room, did the patient quickly move from watching television to lying in bed moaning and groaning? Were they in pain one moment, and asking to go smoke a cigarette the next? These behaviors don't support someone who is in acute pain.

Tweaking—Especially common for patients who abuse methamphetamine, "tweaking" is the way health professionals describe a patient's difficulty focusing, dilated pupils, and jerky body movements.

The importance of a comprehensive assessment procedure and tools to do the job well is stressed throughout this book. While nursing initial assessment tools are effective in identifying some difficult patients, there is room for improvement. Organizations need to develop solutions for integrating the screening of patients' cognitive function into day-to-day procedures. Without examining this critical piece of the assessment procedure, facilities will continue its current struggle to identify their truly difficult patients.

Chapter 4

CASE MANAGEMENT FOR THE DIFFICULT PATIENT

CHAPTER 4

Case Management for the Difficult Patient

In any discussion about case management for the difficult patient populations described in this chapter, one must recognize that the key is developing a consistent approach. It is essential that your approach include a thorough assessment, early intervention when possible, and communication with the patient, families, and community resources.

These are difficult patient populations for whom there are no easy answers. Proactive management of any sort will, at worst, reduce staff frustration and, at best, reduce the utilization of human and financial resources while also improving patient outcomes.

Elderly presenting in the emergency department

As the numbers of elderly continue to grow nationally, so grows the elderly patient population in our health care facilities. This population is associated with complex issues, including assessment, inpatient care, and disposition. In order to appropriately address each of these factors, hospitals must equip themselves with the appropriate knowledge and resources—easily said, but not so easily done.

The elderly patient who accesses the health care system today is likely to have multiple medical and social issues. These appear to increase in direct proportion to age. The complexity of these issues often goes undetected until such time as they require emergency care and/or admission to an acute care facility.

Considerations for the loved ones

A significant number of emergency department (ED) visits by the elderly are for either exacerbation of chronic conditions or traumatic injuries often associated with falls. Although they require the appropriate emergent assessment and interventions, these visits often result in a realization, on the part of family members, that their loved one has reached a point at which current living arrangements and treatment options must be reassessed.

Anyone who has ever been faced with such decisions recognizes how difficult they can be. The degree of difficulty is often compounded if the patient's children no longer live in the area. Their increase in awareness is often accompanied by guilt and anger. They are faced with the reality of their parent's declining health and perhaps their own mortality. It may also be at this point that family members are suddenly forced to interact with a health care system they are not familiar with.

In the presence of all these factors, it should come as no surprise that the family's and the patient's stress and anger levels become evident to all who encounter them. Their demands and their anger reflect their inability to appropriately process and deal with the issues at hand: the care and long-term prognosis of their loved one.

Interaction with the patients and families who are struggling with these issues is emotionally demanding and fraught with the potential for misunderstanding. In the midst of anger, confusion, and often dysfunction, health care professionals and facilities are expected to provide safe care and arrange for the optimum disposition or placement. More often than not, we must also educate families about complex disease processes, available resources, and the complex rules and regulations associated with Medicare.

In order to do this, it is essential that we conduct an accurate assessment of the elderly patient. As we discussed in Chapter 3, your assessment must not be limited to a physical assessment of the patient's current status. It must also assess his or her mental status and their social situation, including his or her need, willingness, and ability to provide self-care or to be cared for.

Assessment needs when caring for the elderly patient

As discussed, there are a number of assessment needs when caring for the elderly patient. This will allow for their safe inpatient management and proper disposition. It also enhances the ability to "case manage" this patient population more effectively.

While many would disagree, the appropriate time to begin a comprehensive assessment of this patient population may be while the patient is still in the emergency department, since a significant portion of this population accesses the hospital through these doors.

Although emergency department staff are busy, facilities that develop an appropriate protocol for assessment of the issues we have discussed may find that they are better able to deal with these patients and may ultimately experience less stress when encountering this patient population and their families.

This early focus on a comprehensive assessment is supported by the Joint Commission on Accreditation of Healthcare Organization's (JCAHO) standards regarding the "Continuum of Care." The goal of this set of standards is to "define, shape, and sequence the following processes and activities to maximize coordination of care." These guidelines identify prehospitalization through discharge care and communication issues.

Aside from meeting a JCAHO standard, following this process will enhance communication and optimize the potential for improved outcomes. Obtaining information early in the hospital encounter allows for early establishment of the plan of care.

Developing a plan of care

Often misunderstood, the plan of care does not always have to include admission to an acute care facility. In many instances, the most appropriate plan may include disposition back home with additional care resources, or admission directly to a long- term care facility. This type of plan requires extensive communication and the presence of a discharge planner in the ED. It may also require short-stay admission after hours or on weekends.

Short-stay (observation status) admissions and "three-midnight" rule

Two of the most misunderstood rules ever promulgated by Center for Medicare & Medicaid Services (CMS) have to do with "observation status" and the "three-midnight" rule.

It has been my experience that even the most seasoned nurse manager may not fully understand the rules pertaining to "status." Simply put, patients who come into the hospital for acute care fall into two categories: inpatient and outpatient.

Thirty years ago, it was simple. If they came to the hospital, they were admitted as inpatients unless they were seen in and dismissed from the ED. Then came outpatient procedures and treatment—thus the terms "inpatient" and "outpatient." Then came the 23-hour rule, which stated that the patient was not considered "inpatient" until after the 24th hour. Then came the rule about "observation status," which says a patient can be hospitalized for several days and still not be considered an "inpatient."

Although the "observation" versus "inpatient" rule affects reimbursement and is fraught with the potential for fraud and abuse if misapplied, the real problem is the lack of understanding by physicians and the public.

Many physicians have great difficulty assigning "status," as they feel it is an administrative duty, and not a patient care issue. In addition, it is not reasonable that physicians be expected to understand the utilization criteria on which status is based. In order to assist in the appropriate status order, some institutions have created admission algorithms for the physician to use (see Figure 4.1).

| Figure 4.1 | | **Status Order** | |

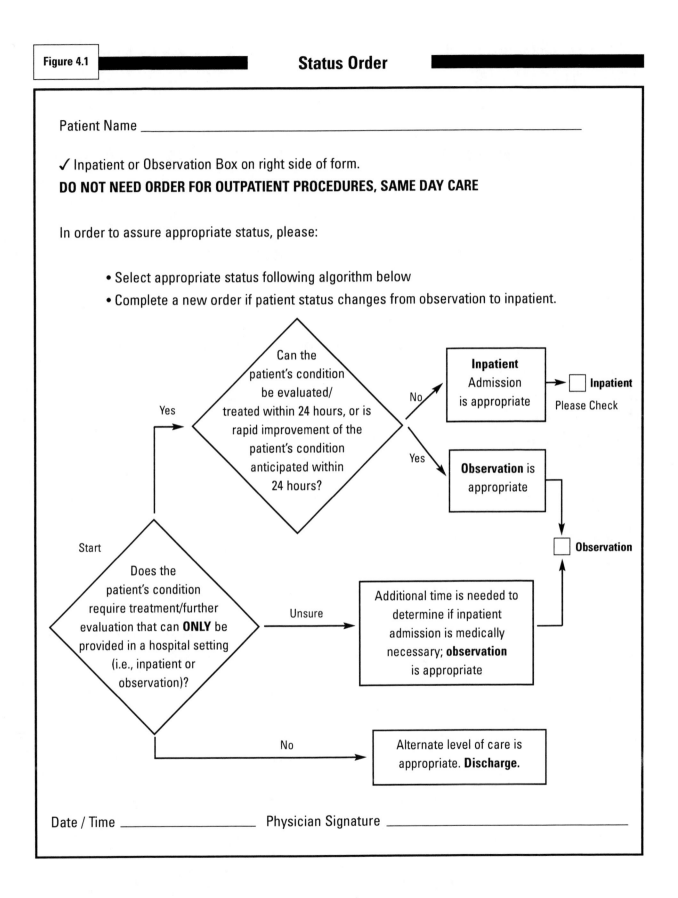

Patient Name _____

✓ Inpatient or Observation Box on right side of form.
DO NOT NEED ORDER FOR OUTPATIENT PROCEDURES, SAME DAY CARE

In order to assure appropriate status, please:

- Select appropriate status following algorithm below
- Complete a new order if patient status changes from observation to inpatient.

Can the patient's condition be evaluated/treated within 24 hours, or is rapid improvement of the patient's condition anticipated within 24 hours?

Yes

No → **Inpatient** Admission is appropriate → ☐ **Inpatient** Please Check

Yes → **Observation** is appropriate

☐ **Observation**

Start

Does the patient's condition require treatment/further evaluation that can **ONLY** be provided in a hospital setting (i.e., inpatient or observation)?

Unsure → Additional time is needed to determine if inpatient admission is medically necessary; **observation** is appropriate

No → Alternate level of care is appropriate. **Discharge.**

Date / Time _____ Physician Signature _____

This tool provides a clear, simple rationale for decision-making. Administrative adjustments may be made using an additional form (see Figure 4.2).

Figure 4.2 ▓▓▓▓▓▓▓▓ **Administrative Status Change Form** ▓▓▓▓▓▓▓▓

Patient Name: _____

ADMINISTRATIVE STATUS CHANGE FORM FOR
COMMERCIAL PAYERS

This form is completed by the Clinical Resource Coordinator (CRC) in response to a commercial payers or DSHS request for Inpatient or Observation Status based on intensity of service and severity of illness.

❏ **Inpatient**

❏ **Observation**

❏ **SDC (Same Day Care)**

❏ **Psych Partial Day Hospitalization**

CRC Signature:_____ Date: _____

For retrospective and concurrent Administrative Status Changes cc Physician

---

The status issue becomes even more significant when dealing with patients and families of the elderly. Having since been adopted by most third-party payers, this rule arose primarily as a result of Medicare/Medicaid reimbursement. However, most people fail to understand how one can spend the night, or several nights, in a hospital and not be considered an inpatient, particularly among other patients who may be inpatients.

Status and long-term care placement

Status becomes a significant issue when long-term care placement is required. Under the current rules, a Medicare patient may be eligible for admission to a skilled nursing facility for up to 100 days of "rehabilitation" following "three midnights" of inpatient hospitalization.

The qualifying stay must be an inpatient status, and the individual must be capable of participating in therapy. Although this sounds easy, families do not understand this benefit and see it merely as a mechanism by which they can reduce out-of-pocket expenses.

Unfortunately, many physicians feel obligated to admit patients solely for the purpose of obtaining "three midnights." Not only is this fraudulent, but the patients often fail to meet the necessary criteria for inpatient status, leaving the family upset and the hospital without the ability to bill the full amount.

Discharge planner in the emergency department

The placement of a discharge planner in the ED, along with targeted education for families and physicians, can reduce both the frequency of these types of admissions and the family's dissatisfaction. It also provides for a more appropriate use of available hospital beds. The discharge planner should make every effort to place individuals in the appropriate care setting directly from the ED when possible.

Fall precautions

In the United States, one in three adults age 65 or older falls each year. Falls are the leading cause of injury deaths among people 65 years and older, with 60% of those deaths occurring in individuals age 70 and older. Among older adults, falls are the most common cause of injuries and trauma-related hospitalization. Fractures are the most serious health outcome associated with falls. Approximately 3% of falls result in fractures, with the most common being fractures of the pelvis, hip, femur, vertebrae, humerus, hand, forearm, leg, and ankle.

For adults age 65 and older, 60% of falls occur at home, 30% in public places, and 10% in health care facilities. Although we will focus primarily on falls in health care institutions, assessment of fall risks should carry over into home and public settings because this can reduce the greatest number of hospitalizations, injuries, and deaths. This is particularly relevant, since the greatest predictor of future falls is the occurrence of previous falls.

Falls are among the most common incidents in health care facilities. Some reports would support fall rates for hospitalized patients of 0.6 to 2.9 falls annually per bed. Long-term care falls are slightly higher, at 0.6 to 3.6 falls annually per bed. For adults age 65 years and older, the total cost of falls injuries in 1994 was an estimated $20.2 billion dollars.

Most institutionally based fall prevention programs incorporate the identification of individuals at risk for falls. The starting point is the history taking, which occurs during the initial assessment. Many facilities have developed their own fall risk scoring system, which generally incorporates history of falls, types of medications taken, ability to ambulate without assistance, mental status, and medical conditions.

One of the most comprehensive fall prevention programs is that of the Veterans Administration, available on their National Center for Patient Safety Web site at: *http://www.patientsafety.gov/FallPrev/Technology.html*. This Web site offers a comprehensive review of a total fall risk program and is available for use by any institution.

The confused elderly patient

As discussed in Chapter 1, a growing number of adults age 65 and older are found to be confused. Although clearly a medical management issue at home, this population becomes increasingly problematic when taken out of a familiar environment and placed in an institutional setting, such as an acute or long-term care facility.

Every effort must be made to ensure that these patients are adequately assessed and that steps are taken to prevent injury from falls, as previously discussed, wandering and elopement, or the host of other risks they may face, including the following:

- Aspiration
- Medication errors
- A medically induced worsening of their confusion

Every effort must be made to communicate with this vulnerable population and their families to accurately assess their risk and to solicit assistance in their management during hospitalization.

Identification of specific needs, habits, communication styles, response to medications, and verbal cues will decrease the likelihood of negative outcomes.

Frequent checks, accompanied by offers to toilet, or provide hydration, nourishment, and reassurance, may reduce the patient's anxiety and accompanying agitation. Systems to prevent patients from wandering may also be of benefit. These may include bed alarms, wander alarms that trigger when a patients exits or attempts to exit a particular door, or controlled access units.

Managing immigrant/migrant patients effectively

The primary focus of management of the immigrant/migrant population is to ensure that we as health care professionals can appropriately meet their needs. In order to do this, we must embrace the concept of cultural competency.

Although many facilities in border states have embraced this concept out of necessity, facilities in other areas have not. Many difficulties can arise from failing to provide culturally competent care, including the environment fraught with the potential for miscommunication, lack of informed consent, and a genuine mistrust on the part of patients, their families, and the health care community.

In caring for your immigrant/migrant population you must first recognize that this population cannot be lumped into one group. The melting pot called the United States continues to receive immigrants from around the globe in increasing numbers. It is essential that health care professionals develop a framework by which to meet their needs.

Language and interpretation issues

Language may be one of the most critical aspects of providing culturally competent care. There are numerous resources available to assist in translation. These include telephonic translations services such as AT&T Language Line and Cyracom International, local fee-for-service interpreters, and hospital-based interpreters.

Although family members may be used in emergencies, it is recommended that alternative methods of translation be implemented for routine use. If your facility has a particularly large non-English–speaking population, you would be well served to recruit health care professionals who speak the prevalent language. Staff must not, however, be allowed to foster the concept that "they are in our country so they should learn English." This will certainly lead to dissatisfaction on the part of the staff and the patients.

Most health care facilities are better served if they formalize their process for requesting interpreter services. This allows for prescheduling and follow-up to ensure the availability of the appropriate interpreter and the correct location. It also provides a mechanism by which to track utilization patterns and billing issues (see Figure 4.3).

Curbing the financial strains

This population often lacks the financial resources necessary to obtain transportation; phone service; or other necessities such as personal hygiene products, adequate nutrition, and proper housing. This reality not only puts them at greater risk for disease and/or trauma, it also leads them to place health care in general, and preventive health care more specifically, at a lower priority. Add to this their cultural beliefs regarding health care and it is much easier to understand their difficulty with accessing and reluctance to access health care in situations other than emergencies.

The immigrant/migrant population is very successful in tapping into community, state, and federal resources. When this occurs, their lack of understanding of the system sometimes leads to overuse of emergency departments for primary care and a failure on the part of the immigrant patients to establish a relationship with a primary care provider.

Figure 4.3 ████████████ **Interpreter Request Form** ████████████

To: Polylang Translation Services
Phone: 425.455.5158
Fax: 425.455.4946

From: Overlake Hospital Medical Center
Social Services
Phone: 425.688.5261
Fax: 425.688.5009

Language Needed: _____

Patient's Name: _____

Patient's Phone Number: _____

Is patient covered by Medicaid (DSHS)? ❏ Yes   ❏ No   ❏ Unknown

Date needed	Time	Length of time

Interpreter preference: _____

Gender preference? ❏ Male ❏ Female

Location of appointment: _____

Person requesting interpreter: _____

The information contained in this facsimile communication is privileged and/or confidential information intended only for the use of the entity named above. If the reader of this cover page is not the intended recipient, you are hereby notified that any dissemination, distribution, or copying of this communication or the information contained in this communication is strictly prohibited. If you have received this communication in error, please immediately notify us by telephone and mail this facsimile to Overlake Hospital Medical Center, 3345 116th Ave. NE, Bellevue, WA 98004

Source: Overlake Hospital Medical Center

Providing a safe environment

The primary goal of cultural competency is to provide a safe environment for these patients by becoming aware of situations and settings that may make them uncomfortable. A mother having to explain some sort of sexual or menstrual dysfunction through translation by a small child is an example. I know of no culture in which this type of situation would be anything but uncomfortable, yet this occurs daily in many facilities.

Focus on understanding. Entering into a situation where you may understand cultural bias and misunderstandings will allow for some degree of flexibility in perceptions and delivery of care. Understand that the presenting complaint may not necessarily be what is really wrong. Trust is not developed overnight. To be thrust into a situation where everyone is different than you would make even the best of us mistrustful.

Acknowledge differences. I am often amazed at how many immigrants are quick to adopt the ways of North Americans, including a functional command of the language, yet those of us who deal with a particular population on a regular basis often fail to learn even the basics of their culture or language.

When delivering culturally competent care, it is important that health care professionals:

- Know where the patient was born and any implications his or her place of birth may have on health care.

- Know what language the patient speaks at home. Even if a patient has some skills in English as a second language, caution must be taken in assessing of their level of comprehension.

- Know the patient's dietary habits, and/or requirements. These may be situational or cultural.

- Know that even if a health care professional does not embrace their belief system, he or she still must understand it.

- Know the patient's religion. Knowledge of particular religions and associated restrictions or requirements will reduce the likelihood of misunderstanding and increase compliance with proposed treatment.

- Determine how the immigrant patient's culture affects their emotional state.

- Obtain information regarding the patient's level of independence within the community.

- Know the patient's support system and how his or her culture may affect ability to access these vital networks.

- Develop relationships with cultural community resources so that appropriate referrals may be made.

- Solicit information from patients on how health issues may be handled in their homes.

- Allow patients to teach the staff their language and culture.

When dealing with this population, it is important to anticipate cultural and communication problems and be proactive in your approach to dealing with them. If problems do arise, communication becomes increasingly important. Use of a translator in these circumstances is best done in person with someone you trust. The translator's ability to translate without interpretation becomes essential.

Managing the effects of caring for the uninsured

It is important to note that the uninsured are not necessarily a specific group of patients. This population also includes the elderly, immigrant/migrants, substance abusers, and mental health patients. The fact that they are uninsured only compounds the problems that the health care community encounters when dealing with these patients.

Reflecting on the principles of your organization

The first step in addressing this issue is to reflect on the mission and founding principles of your organization. Many health care workers confuse an organization's not-for-profit status with a commitment to provide unlimited charity care. Although some organizations exist for exactly that purpose, most do not. Hospitals and health care facilities must remain vigilant in how they manage their financial resources in order to continue to meet their mission because uncompensated care affects all health care providers, including for-profit institutions. It accounted for $21 billion dollars of lost revenues in 2001, and that number continues to grow.

As with the elderly, it is essential to provide a thorough assessment and early intervention. Formalized case management programs that provide for monitoring and oversight, although costly, may prove beneficial in the long run. This is particularly true of individuals who do not follow through with attempts to refer them to community resources. We must be aware that many uninsured are not concerned with the impact another bad debt may have on their current financial situation. It then becomes incumbent on us to shepherd these individuals through the system.

Many urban areas have organizations that will, for a percentage of collected charges, facilitate the process of applying for available funded coverage. Since this is often a complex process, it may be worth the expense to allow them to do so. In smaller communities and/or facilities, it may prove beneficial to assign the task to one person, who then becomes the subject matter expert. They will have developed relationships with the respective agencies and an in-depth understanding of the particular rules and regulations pertaining to coverage issues.

Collecting fees from patients

A growing trend among hospitals that are faced with overcrowding of EDs and loss of revenue associated with uncompensated care is to collect or attempt to collect fees from patients at the time of their visits. The organizations hope that, by collecting fees from the uninsured at the time of service, they may reduce inappropriate utilization of facilities. Although technically legal, organizations must exercise caution so that they avoid violation of Emergency Medical Treatment and Active Labor Act (EMTALA) rules and any negative fallout that may be associated with such a practice.

It is critical that health care providers recognize that this patient population is hypersensitive to the perception that they will be treated differently than paying customers. This often leads to increased demands and anger on the part of the patients and their families. If this becomes an issue, staff should remain focused on providing care and should not become defensive.

Facing the challenges of the chronically mentally ill and substance abusers

A systematic approach to dealing with the chronically mentally ill and substance abusers is essential for all health care facilities. These patients, who frequently fall into the category of uninsured, demand financial and emotional resources to a degree that stresses many organizations. Many facilities have inpatient psychiatric or substance abuse units and may be more adept at dealing with patient and family issues. However, a greater number do not.

For any facility, it is important to focus on early assessment and intervention. Although the chronically mentally ill and substance abusers do require acute care hospitalization, they are more frequently seen in emergency departments, and a disposition is made. In the instances where there is an inpatient psychiatric unit, they may be admitted there. Again, the majority of hospitals do not have inpatient treatment options for this patient population.

The need for crisis intervention with the mentally ill can result in an inordinate demand on staff resources during peak census times in an ED. In institutions where there may be a clinical social worker/crisis intervention specialist, this becomes less of an issue; however, the responsibility for patients, even in this circumstance, remains with the emergency physicians and nurses.

If the facility does not have internal resources, they are at the mercy of community resources and often the County Designated Mental Health Professional (or the person in your state responsible for assessing patients for involuntary commitment).

Establish a resource book

In order to facilitate more rapid disposition, it is recommended that a resource book and contact numbers be developed and maintained. Do not rely too much on published resource guides. They typically have local resources, which are certainly limited in rural areas and increasingly limited in urban areas. With closure of psychiatric units increasing, it is not unusual for EDs to be faced with referrals for both voluntary and involuntary inpatient admissions that require transportation across county lines or even across state lines. Therefore, the greater your resource list, the greater likelihood that you will have an appropriate and timely disposition.

Develop a plan of care with a mental health professional

For the chronically mentally ill who are seen in your facility's ED on a frequent basis, it may prove beneficial to develop a plan of care with their respective attending mental health professionals. This will allow for a better understanding of their conditions, and may facilitate acute stabilization and referral to the provider's office for an outpatient assessment. Since the mental health provider is more familiar with the patient, he or she may determine that there is not a need for inpatient hospitalization, or may have a greater list of resources from which to draw.

The chronically mentally ill may lack family support, in that they have either disengaged from the family, or more often than not, their families have, over time, become frustrated with the demands that have been placed on them. When dealing with both the supportive and nonsupportive families, staff should

- allow them to verbalize
- remain nonjudgmental
- refrain from criticizing the patient's condition or lifestyle

Drug abusers and drug seekers

One of the most difficult patient populations for staff to deal with are the drug abusers/drug seekers, who are flooding the EDs of both urban and rural hospitals. As with the mentally ill, resources are scarce. Although there is little we can do to prevent drug-associated trauma, facilities can address and effectively deal with drug seekers.

Many facilities and providers feel pressured to prescribe narcotics, even in the presence of no objective findings. Part of this is due to the focus on pain as the "fifth vital sign," and part of it is because there is an understanding that it is very difficult to objectify pain.

Record accurate history and complete a thorough examination

There is no definitive test to diagnose the type, nature, and degree of pain an individual may experience. What can be done, however, is to record an accurate history and complete a thorough examination. Part of the history should be a review of old medical records if available. Review of these documents may reveal a pattern of visits for a variety of complaints or maybe just one. Typically the pattern will include periods of increased frequency followed by periods of reduced or no visits. This is a typical pattern because the drug-seeking patient, in an effort to not raise suspicion, may alternate treatment facilities.

What providers should remember, despite their frustration and the demand that this population places on a facility's human and financial resources, is that the majority of these patients are addicted. You may or may not agree that addiction is a disease. However, you cannot argue that addiction requires treatment if there is to be any hope of recovery. Acknowledgment of addiction is not an argument to indiscriminately prescribe narcotics or other controlled drugs. It is the recognition that a plan of care must be developed to help these patients.

"Drug-seeker lists"

Many institutions have unofficial lists of drug seekers. The Health Insurance Portability and Accountability Act of 1996 (HIPAA) has lead some to discontinue the practice, which is not always the most reliable method for obtaining accurate information.

Providers must remember that HIPAA does not prohibit communication between providers involved in the treatment of a patient. This is important in communicating between facilities. It is also important should you decide, as many facilities do, to create plans of care for patients who frequent a facility with complaints of pain.

Plan of care

Many institutions develop, with the assistance of primary care providers, a plan of care for prescription drug abusers and seekers. This allows for a continuity of care and management of an individual's medication use. It will also reduce the likelihood that a patient will supplement his or her prescribed pain medication with visits to EDs. This does require time and willingness on the part of primary care physicians; however, as there becomes an increased focus on prescribing patterns, many physicians have found lists such as these to be of benefit.

Finally, health care providers and facilities must determine whether they will seek to prosecute individuals who fraudulently obtain controlled substances. This takes time and a consistent approach by the providers within a facility. In the end; however, when faced with the consequences of their addiction and the actions they have taken, many patients will seek the appropriate treatment.

Chapter 5

RISK MANAGEMENT FOR PATIENT VIOLENCE

CHAPTER 5

Risk Management for Patient Violence

Going to work shouldn't be a fearful experience. Yet workplace violence has increased over the years, and nurses are among the many employees who are at risk of being physically and verbally abused.

Between 1993 and 1999, 429,100 nurses were victims of violent crime in the workplace annually, according to a Bureau of Justice Statistics special report. That is an average of 21.9 attacks for every 1,000 nurses. In comparison, physicians experienced 71,300 attacks, or 16.2 for every 1,000 doctors.

The American Nurses Association (ANA), which has been tracking assaults on nurses, reports that workplace violence against ANA members has steadily increased over the past few years. The Occupational Safety and Health Administration (OSHA) confirms the rising rate of assaults and reports that the risk of job-related violence against health care and social workers is, at present, higher than for any other field.

To protect staff, organizations need to adopt a zero-tolerance policy against abuse or threats of abuse. Nurses should never have to accept violence in the workplace as "part of their job," even if they work in the emergency department (ED) or a psychiatric facility.

Ensuring a safe workplace for staff

To promote a safe workplace, staff and their nurse managers should work with administrators to implement the following strategies:

Violence management training

Provide violence management training to nurses and other staff members in which they learn how to diffuse potentially dangerous situations. Self-protection is a critical skill that isn't taught in most nursing schools.

Develop policies and procedures

Develop specific policies and procedures to address violence. Your policies must address violence in the workplace, management of psychiatric patients, and security policies. Adopt a "show of force" procedure. In this policy, at the first sign of a potentially violent situation, a nurse pages security for a show of force, rather than waiting until the patient acts out. Nurses are encouraged to de-escalate the situation verbally in the presence of security rather than managing the situation on their own.

Develop a method for alerting staff of a patient's history of violence

Alert other medical staff if a patient has a history of violence. Experts consider this the single most important predictor of violent behavior. If a patient has struck out before at staff, make sure staff caring for the patient know the patient may have violent tendencies.

Educate staff about panic buttons and a violence code

Have panic buttons and establish an emergency code for nurses to summon help. Also ensure that your facility has a clear protocol for responding to emergency codes that signal patient violence.

Schedule workplace assessments

Does your facility hold regular workplace assessments to address the issue of workplace violence? If not, plan to meet on a regular basis with representatives from nursing, security, the union, and other relevant departments to discuss how your facility can implement and improve on current security measures. If violence does occur, assess how such a situation could have been prevented and take action to ensure that it won't happen again.

Encourage staff to report incidents

Be supportive of staff who do encounter workplace violence. Ensure that they report and document incidents and receive all necessary treatment, including counseling. Never make the injured party feel the violence was his or her fault or that they could have prevented the incident.

In addition, Robert Siciliano, a Boston-based professional speaker, personal security consultant, and president of three security-related companies, has these suggestions for keeping your workplace a safe environment for staff to work:

Assess OSHA compliance

The Occupational Safety & Health Administration (OSHA) has established guidelines for preventing workplace violence that include, but are not limited to, incorporating ongoing training to respond to crisis, cooperation between frontline employees and management, determining workplace hazards by analyzing potential isolation areas and risk factors, and having a plan of action to deal with threats, violence, and weapons. Is your organization noncompliant in any of these areas? Work with administrators to make sure your policies, procedures, training, and equipment are all in compliance.

Identify employee-specific responsibilities

Make sure staff learn their assigned duties and comply with your established security program guidelines. Ensure that staff are involved in ongoing procedures, committees, inspections, reporting, and dissemination of information.

Complete a premise security needs assessment

Does your organization have the security equipment needed to maintain a safe environment for staff? Assess your need for security guards, metal detectors, pass keys, alarm systems, panic buttons, cell phones, proper lighting, and centralized radios. A central office to respond to distress calls is essential. Security cameras and curved mirrors assist in remote areas.

Establish contact with law enforcement

Unfortunately, law enforcement's job is usually to respond after a crisis. It is important, however, to create a relationship with local authorities and make them fully aware of the facility's layout. Properly trained security guards can usually diffuse violent situations, whether by nonviolent means or with force.

Educate staff about the buddy system

Pairing staff can offset the chances of being overpowered by a violent patient. Elevators, stairwells, parking garages, home visits, and isolated areas are all potentially threatening situations for staff who are alone.

Educate staff about potential weapons

Not only is jewelry a potential target for thieves, it is a strangulation hazard. Carry only essential identification and cash. Beware of improvised weaponry in the form of surgical tools, keys, pens, or other items.

Factors that contribute to violent behavior

There are countless reasons a patients' behavior could become violent. However, some common factors are known to contribute to violent behavior. These include:

- Not enough staff
- High-volume units or busy times of day
- Invading a patient's personal space
- Use of restraints on an already combative patient
- Staff not experienced in handling aggressive patients

Nurse managers need to work with hospital administration, security, and labor unions to make changes, monitor and document incidents, and assess whether current department actions are effective. Possible solutions to implement include:

- Adding staff during busy seasons/time of day
- Having clinicians on each shift trained in violence prevention

- Holding training programs to teach staff how to protect themselves and deal with patient violence

- Considering installing panic buttons in vulnerable departments

- Considering use of metal detectors

- Improving lighting and video surveillance

- Making it mandatory for all staff to wear ID badges

- Implementing protocols on how your hospital handles threats, harassment, and violence

De-escalating anger in difficult patients

Anger can present itself in many different ways within your organization. Patients' complaints and criticism, disgruntled former employees, and frustrated families are just a few ways. It is essential that your staff be equipped with techniques for preventing that anger from escalating into a violent confrontation.

Staff need to recognize that anger de-escalation begins by maintaining the proper distance (3 to 6 feet) from patients who have a history of violence or who exhibit aggressive behavior. Nurses should then project a calm attitude and active listening skills, acknowledging that the patient is upset and asking for their recommendations to correcting the problem.

Many nurses mistakenly take an irate patient's behavior personally. Part of a training session on workplace violence should include techniques nurses can use to properly manage their own frustration and anger when dealing with difficult patients and stressful situations.

Verbal techniques for de-escalating angry patients

Listen to the patient and respond with empathy
Listen to what the patient is saying without interrupting and try to validate his or her feelings. Most patients calm down once they are allowed to vent their frustrations or concerns. Interrupting and/or denying a patient's feelings can make the situation worse. When the patient pauses, calmly say something like, "I understand you are upset." Remain nonjudgmental, show empathy, and let the patient know you want to address his or her concerns.

Be aware of your paraverbals

Paraverbals include the tone, volume, and rate used when addressing the angry patient. Remember, an upset patient is beginning to lose rational thought, so he or she isn't focused on your actual words. A nurse's tone of voice should be calm, and nurses should avoid sounding impatient, disgusted, or sarcastic. A nurse should speak clearly and slowly in a moderate tone. Speaking too fast or too slowly conveys agitation and loss of control. By speaking calmly and clearly, you are more likely to be heard.

Use the patient's name

Use his or her name respectfully when talking with a patient. This can help diffuse the patient's anger, and convey to them that you are genuinely interested in resolving his or her concerns.

Set non-negotiable limits

Give patients clear choices and consequences for their actions. For example, to a verbally abusive patient you might say, "If you refrain from using profanity, we can discuss your concerns. If not, this conversation is ended." Choices need to be clear, concise, and enforceable.

Memorize The Four Ds

When dealing with angry patients, remember The Four Ds:

- **Disarming:** Engage in conversation with a patient only after he or she has "cooled down."

- **Diverting:** Shift the focus from the patient's angry behavior to the issues behind the angry behavior. This technique works well with "chronic complainers" who need to have their negative attitudes removed before any progress can be made.

- **Diffusing:** Remain calm and refuse to escalate angry behavior by reinforcing it with verbal retaliation or aggressive body language.

- **Deflecting:** Use silence selectively as a means of ignoring verbal attacks.

Nonverbal techniques for de-escalating angry patients

Your nonverbal communication techniques are the most important aspect of your de-escalation strategies. Studies show, when in a rational state of mind, body language conveys about 55% of our message and verbal communication only about 10%. When you are de-escalating patient anger, your body language is communicating more to your angry patient than your words are.

Here are some tips for making sure your body is saying what it should:

Respect a patient's personal space

Personal space is the area around a person in which he or she feels safe. For most patients, two to three feet should be a safe parameter; it is three to six feet for patients who have a history of exhibiting aggressive behavior. Entering an upset person's personal space can intensify his or her emotions. Remember, an angry patient may already feel he or she is losing control simply by being in the hospital.

Maintaining an open stance

Nurses should slightly turn their body at an angle to the patient while keeping their hands open and in plain view. Angry patients will perceive this stance as less threatening than one where you stand with your hands on your hips, for example. Nurses should also refrain from crossing their arms or pointing fingers, both or which are gestures that can also send out a negative message.

Maintain appropriate eye contact and facial expressions

A nurse's face and eyes convey a direct message to the other patient. Nurses should maintain general eye contact, not stare through the other person. It's important to be aware of cultural habits within your patient population. Some ethnic groups consider it inappropriate to look directly at another person when he or she is upset or being disciplined. A nurse's facial expression should be serious but not angry or fearful. You want to convey concern and control. Nurses do not want their facial expressions to imply that the patient's condition is more serious than the patient believes or that the nurse does not care about their situation.

Chapter 6

MOVING TOWARD A RESTRAINT-FREE FACILITY

CHAPTER 6

Moving Toward a Restraint-Free Facility

Nurses have long walked a fine line when caring for patients who are at risk of harming themselves or others. Creating an environment that offers patients both dignity and safety isn't an easy task. However, it is incumbent upon all health care professionals to take steps to protect their patients and their colleagues.

One of the first methods that comes to mind is restraints.

The changing restraint climate

Restraints, used frequently in the past, have fallen out of favor. Studies and anecdotal evidence have demonstrated that restraint use with all of the difficult patient populations we've discussed in this book was not conclusively effective. In many instances, it resulted in a worsening of agitation, injuries, and even death.

Based on these findings, the Joint Commission on Accreditation of Healthcare Organizations (JCAHO) released standards for restraints in 1996 and revised them in 1999.

Also in 1999, the Centers for Medicare and Medicaid Services (CMS) (formerly known as the Health Care Financing Administration [HCFA]) released its "Patient Rights of Condition of Participation," stating that hospitals had to meet new standards to be approved for and continue participation in Medicare and Medicaid programs.

These guidelines restrict the use of both chemical and physical restraints to situations in which patients are actually a threat to themselves or others. This use of "behavioral restraints" is episodic. It requires immediate physician response and must be frequently monitored.

The use of alternative interventions is required both prior to and during use of physical restraints. Chemical restraint, which is best described as the use of pharmacological agents to control a patient's behavior, is also restricted.

Restraint use has now become very labor intensive, in terms of both staff requirements (applying and monitoring the restraints) and physician involvement (ordering, initial and ongoing assessment, and termination of restraint use).

Every effort must be made to engage the physician in the process because physician involvement is a key component of compliance with current rules and guidelines. Standing order sheets provide a clear template for physicians and need not be complex.

Equally time consuming is dealing with the issue of restraint use when it is either presented by the family or required by patient behaviors. Many families fail to understand why we do not restrain or "tie down" their loved one. They often become angry and threaten future claims or legal action should a fall or injury occur.

Early education and continued communication are the keys to overcoming this potential landmine. Other things to consider when restraints must be applied:

- Staff should communicate, from beginning to end, the rationale for applying restraints

- Staff should also relate which alternatives have been considered and timeframes for restraint use

- Most importantly, staff should follow the policies at your institution and document the entire process

Protecting yourself through documentation

Thorough documentation is one of your organization's best protections against accusations of improper restraint usage and potential litigation. Also, your clear and complete documentation of these episodes will serve as the foundation for quality improvement efforts.

Some organizations choose to record this information in the patient's record, whereas others use a separate restraint log or flowsheet. It is worth reminding your staff that, regardless of the method, documentation must be clear and complete. It is also worth reminding staff that these records do not exist merely for those caring for the patient or other facility personnel. Their documentation can be used as evidence in a court of law.

- Dating entries is not enough. All entries should have a precise time. Without the time, it may be impossible to show that actions were taken in accordance with your policy requirements or federal and state regulatory standards.

- Checklist-style documentation may fall short of offering good clinical justification for using restraints. Regardless of whether your organization uses this style, there must be an acknowledgment that "danger to self and others" is not sufficient explanation. Solid justification should include:

  - A description of the patient's behavior
  - The alternatives to restraints that were tried but were unsuccessful
  - The education efforts attempted, if any

Preparing your staff for a move away from restraints

The use of restraints has always been controversial, and new research shows that restraints can pose a safety risk and should only be utilized only as a last resort. As a result, many medical centers and long-term care facilities have adopted policies aimed at reducing or eliminating the use of patient restraints.

If this concept seems implausible, keep in mind that facilities implement these new procedures slowly, reviewing patients on a case-by-case basis. With the commitment of nursing and hospital leadership, it is possible to eliminate or reduce the use of restraints in both acute and long-term care facilities.

Reduction of restraint use in your facility will be a gradual and systemic process. To begin the process, a facility must have the commitment to restraint reduction from the top administrator down to front-line caregivers.

In nursing school, many nurses learned that restraints were a traditional method of keeping patients safe, as well as a means of preventing combative and agitated patients from harming themselves or others. Nurses need to be shown that, rather than thinking a patient is safe when restrained, he or she can actually be at risk of both injury and loss of human dignity.

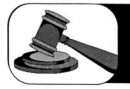

CASE STUDY: A NEW JERSEY HOSPITAL MAKES COMMITMENT TO REDUCE RESTRAINT USE

In 1995, Underwood Memorial Hospital in Woodbury, NJ, made a commitment to reduce restraint usage in their facility. Since that time, they have kept restraint usage below 5%.

Staff leaders credit the following strategies for Underwood Memorial's reduction in restraint usage.

- A very active restraint team composed of nurses from all departments who meet on a monthly basis to review order sheets and conduct random restraint reviews.

- A process for inviting medical vendors onsite to present new products that are alternatives to restraints or products that directly reduce restraint usage. Marla Maybrook, RN, manager of quality improvement at Underwood Memorial, notes the facility will use products on a trial basis in various units. The team is always looking for new ways to improve on its goal of keeping restraint usage to a minimum.

- Acknowledging there may be some patients such as those on ventilators and certain emergency department (ED) cases in which restraint use is still the safest option.

Before a facility can begin to reduce or eliminate restraints, workshops need to be held to address the use of restraints, introduce viable alternatives to restraints, and answer questions and educate staff on the use and dangers of restraints.

Common questions and answers regarding restraint-free policies

When a facility decides to move toward reducing restraints, nurses may question whether this is the best strategy. Common concerns revolve around patient safety and staffing concerns. As a nurse manager, you may hear a variety of questions from concerned staff. Here are some commonly asked questions and answers:

 Will using fewer restraints mean more patient falls?

Studies show that restraints will not keep patients from falling. Falls that occur when someone is not restrained generally result in less injury than falls that happen when the patient is restrained. Facilities that have attempted to release patients from restraints have documented a decrease in falls and fall-related injury.

 Will caring for patients who were previously restrained require that nurses spend more time with these patients?

No. Facilities that have reduced restraints have actually documented a decrease in staff time required to care for previously restrained patients. Untie the Elderly, a not-for-profit training and consulting company specializing in long-term care issues, has documentation available that shows patients who are restrained require more time from nurses or nursing assistants than do similarly impaired residents who are not restrained. Remember, when a patient is in restraints, nurses are required to check on him or her every 15 minutes, as well as provide documentation.

Is the concept of reducing restraints even feasible in light of the nursing shortage?

 Yes. Many hospitals and long-term care facilities have moved to this model without increasing staffing. Studies show that it takes more nursing time to care for a patient in restraints. Also keep in mind that moving toward a restraint-free facility does not mean releasing all patients from restraints and hoping for the best outcome. Facilities that implement these strategies do so on a case-by-case basis. When a restraint is removed, a restraint alternative is used, and for some patients, nursing staff may decide that some form of restraint is still the only viable option for keeping the patient safe.

Can restraint reduction actually work in an acute-care setting? Can it also work in a long-term care facility?

Yes. Both acute-care and long-term facilities have successfully become restraint-free. Special care units for the cognitively impaired have reduced or eliminated restraints without seeing any increase in behavioral problems or injuries. Facilities that have implemented restraint-free policies have reported higher satisfaction rates among both staff and patients.

Strategies for educating your staff about a restraint reduction program

Hold a facility-wide orientation. Use this opportunity to introduce your plans to reduce or eliminate restraints. Provide supportive literature and a summary of state and federal regulations. Follow it with smaller workshops that teach nurses and other staff about restraint alternatives and how they can incorporate them into patient care.

Designate a unit to pilot test your plan. Designate a specific unit in your facility to begin implementing a restraint-free program.

Re-introduce de-escalation training. Educate nurses about how to interact with patients who become agitated, confused, or combative. The success of your program will depend on your ability to improve the following:

- Staff members' sensitivity to patient's rights
- Verbal and nonverbal de-escalation skills
- Safe physical management techniques

Incorporate your bedside care providers into the process. Encourage your nurses and other staff members to brainstorm ideas and be an active part of the process to make their unit free of restraints.

Design a process for assessing your progress. Organize an interdisciplinary restraint review committee that can meet on a regular basis to track the facility's progress, review restraint orders, and determine how you can continue to decrease the use of restraints among patients and improve quality of care.

Alternatives for patients at risk of falling

Facilities who have implemented restraint-free policies have reported a decrease in the number of patient falls, and the severity of injuries to patients who fall as a result of climbing over or through bed rails.

Suggested techniques for alternatives to restraints for the elderly and other at-risk patient populations are as follows:

- Eliminate standard-height beds with rails for patients who are at risk of falling. Facilities have replaced these beds with ones that are low to the floor. If a patient climbs out of bed, he or she will roll onto a padded mat. Low beds also ensure that patients won't hurt themselves as they try to climb through or over bed rails.

- Identify patients who are at risk of falling by affixing a star ("falling star") to their wheel-chairs and outside their rooms to notify staff that they are a fall risk.

- Purchase nonslip slippers and provide them to patients for free.

- Invest in gripper pads, like the ones often used to line cabinets in your home. Putting this type of pad in a patient's wheelchair or bed can reduce the chances of the patient sliding out and falling to the floor.

- Think about where you place bedside commodes. Placing a bedside commode near the patient so it can be easily and safely used when needed may cut down the potential for falls at your facility.

- For patients who are incontinent, set up a care management plan by which the patient is taken to the toilet every two hours when awake. This should reduce the chance that patients will attempt to get to the restroom on his or her own.

- Since nurses have a limited amount of time with each patient, train nurses to ask if there is anything else they can do for a patient before they leave the room.

- Use bed and chair alarms (both built-in and portable) to monitor a patient's movements.

- Hire paid, trained sitters, who are from a health care agency, to sit at the bedside of patients who are at risk of falling.

Alternatives for patients who become anxious

Hospitals across the country are beginning to use highly trained volunteers for inpatient companion-ship and recreational/diversional activities with adult patients. Talk with your hospital volunteer coor-dinator and recreational therapist about the possibility of working with a local volunteer organization to train volunteers to work in your hospital. Volunteers read to patients, play cards, listen to music, and reminisce with older adults. Some hospitals even provide an activity cart within each unit from which volunteers can choose games and books to help them interact with patients. These volunteers have proven to be a godsend to nursing staff, who have only a limited amount of time to spend with each patient.

Planning activities to be held throughout the day and early evening can be especially effective in reducing the effects of "sundowning." *Sundowning* is a term experts have used to describe the period of increased confusion, anxiety, agitation, and disorientation beginning at dusk and continuing throughout the night that affects many Alzheimer's patients. Many facilities have found that a healthy schedule of daytime activities keeps the minds and bodies of patients occupied and discourages afternoon napping, which may contribute to anxiety at dusk and sleeplessness.

Utilize pet therapy in your workplace. Make contact with a volunteer group that offers pet therapy and invite them to your facility at certain times, or, if you have a staff member with a well-trained pet, allow him or her to bring it to work. The calming effects of pets have been widely documented.

Make "confusion bags" an integral part of your unit. These bags are full of things for confused patients to do to keep their hands busy, such as balls of yarn, small handballs, zippers, or any other items that are safe and keeps the patient's mind occupied. These tasks have been shown to reduce patients' level of anxiety.

Utilize music therapy. Music has been shown to have a calming effect on many patients. Keep headphones and radios on hand to use with patients who become anxious or agitated.

Often elderly patients who reside in long-term care facilities don't have family members who live close by. Encourage these distant family members to send photos and a cassette tape with a recording of their voices talking to the patient. Some facilities have found that playing a tape recording of a patient's family talking reduces the patient's anxiety level.

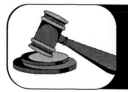

CASE STUDY: NORTH CAROLINA NURSING HOME CREATES ALTERNATIVES FOR PATIENTS PRONE TO PULLING ON TUBES AND CATHETERS

WakeMed, a private, not-for-profit, 758-bed, multifacility health system in Raleigh, NC, initiated an intensive focus on restraint reduction in its acute care and rehabilitation settings. Diane Baggett, director of Medical/Surgical Services, and Fran Powell, supervisor/educator, Urology/Renal Unit, shared some of the following strategies in a report published in the Untie the Elderly newsletter:

- Buy gardening gloves to put on the hands of these at-risk patients. These gloves are large and bulky and make it difficult for the patient to grasp the tube. If they can still manage to pull at the tube, put a small foam ball inside the palm of the glove to make squeezing their hands more challenging. The patients loved this strategy, because they could now squeeze the ball and exercise their hands, providing a diversion.

- For male patients with Foley catheters in place, boxer shorts were used in addition to the standard leg band. The boxer shorts hid the catheter from view, eliminating the patient's temptation to pull on the catheter. This strategy also works with patients who have G-tubes. Once applied, an abdominal binder, restricts the patient's ability to remove the tube.

Alternatives for patients who become agitated

First and foremost, encourage nurses to request tests to rule out the possibility of infection. If a patient with a neurological condition such as Alzheimer's has a sudden cognitive or behavioral change, one of the first things to consider is an acute illness.

With neurological diseases, you don't see abrupt changes in a patient's condition, so a sudden change signifies that something else is happening. Especially if patients are nonverbal, the only cues that they are in pain may be their acting out.

Recent medical studies have shown that a whiff of lavender or exposure to bright light might be enough to relieve some of dementia's most disturbing symptoms, including agitation, aggression, depression, and sleep disturbances.

In the December 7, 2002, issue of the *British Medical Journal*, Alistair Burns, professor of old-age psychiatry at the University of Manchester, released the results of three studies showing that the use of aromatherapy, specifically lemon balm and lavender oil, reduced agitation and improved the patients' quality of life. The oils were either inhaled or applied to a patient's skin.

Bright light, known to be effective in treating seasonal affective disorder, was also used in the studies. The treatment involved dementia patients sitting in front of a specially designed light box that gives off a much brighter light than normal office or home lighting. Studies have shown that full-spectrum light can also reduce the effects of sundowning.

Alternative for dementia patients: validation therapy

A technique that is being used more with patients who have dementia is validation therapy. The idea behind validation therapy is to join patients on their mental journeys to the past instead of vainly trying to snap them back to the present. The result is better communication with less frustration and agitation for both patients and nurses.

Facilities that have embraced validation therapy provide patients with props and furnishings that signify a place in their life that was comfortable for them. Many patients enjoy rocking a doll as they remember taking care of their own children. The idea behind validation therapy is to validate, or accept, the values, beliefs, and "reality" of the dementia patient. Under this method of thinking, no one tells the patient waiting for her husband to pick her up that in reality, her husband is dead and she is in a long-term care facility. Instead, she might be asked about her favorite date or what she plans to wear for the special outing.

If your facility hasn't tried validation therapy, consider holding a workshop for nurses. The training itself provides a solid ground for nurses to better understand the thought process of patients with cognitive impairment.

Chapter 7

Improving Patient and Family Satisfaction in Specific Units

CHAPTER 7

Improving Patient and Family Satisfaction in Specific Units

Some of your difficulties with patients and families may be influenced by the environment fostered by specific departments in your facility. In this chapter we discuss the challenges to patient and family satisfaction that are common in three areas of acute-care facilities—the emergency department (ED), critical care unit (CCU), and the intensive care unit (ICU)—and provide you with proactive strategies for addressing those challenges before they lead to difficulties.

Difficult patients and families in the emergency department

Jackie Delacy, RN, worked for many years as the ED nurse manager in one of northern California's busiest EDs. On any given day, Delacy and her staff would treat gunshot victims, drug overdoses, and a variety of trauma cases. Delacy, who now works as a health care consultant, shares some of the strategies she used to prevent patients from becoming difficult in the ED:

- Train ED nurses to regularly check in with patients. Peeking your head in the door and saying, "We haven't forgotten about you. Can I get you anything while you're waiting?" goes a long way toward keeping patients happy.
- Identify yourself as soon as you enter the examination room. With the steady flow of employees going in and out of the ED, Delacy recommends that all nurses introduce themselves and explain to the patient why they are there: "Hi, Mr. Jones. My name is Sophie. I'm your nurse, and I'm here to take your blood pressure."

- Treat all patients with the same level of respect. Even if a patient suffers from dementia, explain procedures to him or her in the same manner you would use with any other patient. Patients with cognitive impairment can become alarmed when someone comes into a room and immediately begins taking their blood pressure or administering care without explaining his or her actions.

- Talk to all patients in a soothing, reassuring manner, even if you think they don't under-stand.

- Give patients back some of the control. Patients are usually extremely fearful when they come into the ED. Nurses can help allay their fears by engaging them in conversation and then giving a patient choices such as, "In which arm would you like the IV inserted?" This allows the patients to regain some control over his or her care.

Does your ED have a patient representative?

Does your hospital have a patient representative assigned to the ED? If not, consider approaching administrators about the possibility of hiring someone for this position.

Many EDs have staffed this position effectively by using interns from its social work department, qualified volunteers, and even retired nurses.

Patient representatives help ease the load for clinical staff while helping increase patient satisfaction. Patient representatives make the rounds in waiting rooms and patient examination rooms, offering blankets, pillows, wait time information, and coffee and juice as allowed. These representatives can also act as go-betweens when patients have concerns or questions, letting the triage nurse know about concerns before they become complaints.

Hospitals who have implemented a patient representative typically report an increase in their patient satisfaction scores. This is an easy and cost-effective way to assist nursing staff and to let patients and their families know that your hospital is making an extra effort to make this ED visit go as smoothly as possible.

Long wait times and other access issues

One of the most common scenarios faced by ED staff are patients who become angry because of long waits to see a doctor. Although nurses can't reduce a patient's wait time, checking in with patients on a regular basis and apologizing for the long wait can help diffuse their anger.

Susan Keane Baker, a motivational speaker in the health care field, suggests the following changes to your waiting area that may make a patient's or concerned family's wait time more enjoyable or at least more tolerable:

Provide activities. Baker suggests a minimum of eight different magazines reflecting the interests of your patients, books on tape, crossword puzzle pads, stationery for writing letters, and a phone for local calls. Also consider including crayons and coloring books for children.

Offer a library of consumer health books. A local bookstore may provide the library for you in exchange for adding to your waiting area the store's business cards and a sign saying that any of the books can be ordered by phone.

Provide soothing distractions. Display art exhibits by children or "words of wisdom" exhibits by older adults. Think about adding headphones and relaxation tapes, an aquarium, or rocking chairs.

Ensure furnishings are comfortable and refreshments are available. Are the chairs in your waiting room actually comfortable? Keep coffee and water on hand for patients, families, and friends to serve themselves while waiting.

ED TIP: There's nothing worse than feeling ill and not being able to find a parking place in the hospital parking lot. To alleviate this problem, Swedish Hospital in Englewood, CO, offers complimentary valet parking services from 8 a.m. to 5 p.m., Monday through Friday. Valet parking is provided for mothers with babies or small children, senior citizens, and physically challenged patients.

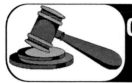

CASE STUDY: NEW MODEL OF NURSING CARE REDUCES ED WAIT TIMES AND IMPROVES PATIENT AND NURSE SATISFACTION

Coney Island Hospital in Brooklyn, NY, has established a new nursing care model that has produced significant results in improving patient care, decreasing ED wait times, and increasing both patient and nurse satisfaction.

The hospital's new Enhanced Continuum of Care (ECC) program gives nurses more time to focus their attention on patients, and less on paperwork. Since ECC has been implemented, the hospital's documentation compliance rate has improved and discharge time for patients has been decreased from more than two hours to 30 minutes.

The work redesign included assigning registered nurses to work in the emergency room to transition patients to the units and help complete paperwork, thus maintaining continuity of care and freeing time for nurses on the general units to spend time with patients and patients' families. The new ED admitting nurse interviews patients and develops a care plan, explains hospital procedures and answers patient questions.

A patient satisfaction study taken before the new care plan showed that 73% of patients thought nurses spent too much time on paperwork. In the most recent survey, only 6% of patients felt the same way.

Another aspect of the ECC takes place at the end of the hospital stay. Special discharge nurses ensure that each patient leaves the hospital expediently. A call is placed to the patient the next day to ensure that all instructions were understood and to get feedback on the overall hospital stay. The personal attention and follow-up call give patients a better impression of the hospital.

One of the priorities of the ECC model was staff satisfaction. Administrators and nurse managers wanted to utilize nurses more efficiently and give them what they wanted—more autonomy and more control over patient management.

Coney Island Hospital involved nurses from all levels and departments in developing the ECC model. One of the items learned from internal surveys and interviews was the nurses' interest in ongoing education. The hospital now offers accredited courses at no cost to nurses. The hospital has also eliminated mandatory overtime, which kept nurses away from their families and increased nurse "burnout."

Nurse turnover at Coney Island has been very low—about 2% to 3% compared with a national average of 6% to 9%. Another benefit was that there were no additional costs involved in implementing the plan, because the hospital redefined certain roles to accommodate the new admission and discharge nurses.

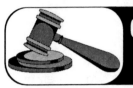 **CASE STUDY: THREE-STEP PROCESS LEADS TO FASTER, MORE EFFICIENT ED VISITS AT NEW JERSEY FACILITY**

Riverview Medical Center in Red Bank, NJ, recently implemented changes to improve access and patient comfort while decreasing wait times in its ED.

Riverview ED staff accomplish this by moving their patients through a three-step process:

1. A nurse now meets every ambulatory patient as he or she walks through the ED doors. This nurse is assisted by a "greeter" who provides help in the ED 24 hours a day and acts as a patient guide, doing everything from making sure the patient's car is valet-parked to providing the latest information or developments to a patient's family.
2. Once the patient's level of need is determined, he or she is registered and then shown to the appropriate area of the ED, either a treatment room in the main ED or a "fastrack" room, where minor injuries and illnesses can be treated promptly.
3. After a preliminary assessment and appropriate testing is conducted, the patient goes to the postprocedure room. There, the test results are reviewed and treatment instructions are given.

Using this new model of care, wait times are reduced, as patients move through the ED more rapidly and treatment rooms open up more quickly for the next patient. Patients are also pleased with the increased communication offered by this new model of care.

Handling intoxicated patients in the ED

Intoxicated patients have long posed a problem for ED staff. Although chronic alcoholics typically don't require emergency medical intervention, they can tie up emergency room beds for hours at a time.

Emergency rooms are required to keep intoxicated patients until their blood alcohol level drops, which can take anywhere from five to 10 hours. Typically the patients don't require treatment, yet emergency room staff must keep them until they are sober enough to be released. Since emergency rooms often see several thousand patients a year whose sole problem is intoxication, chronic alcoholics can create a strain on already overcrowded emergency rooms.

To address this dilemma, many emergency rooms across the United States are examining whether they can provide a more suitable care alternatives to intoxicated patients.

In San Francisco, CA, an Emergency Room Diversion Task Force, which is composed of members of the Board of Supervisors and representatives from the public and private sectors, addressed the problem of overcrowded emergency rooms by introducing the McMillan Stabilization Project. This project is intended to free up emergency room hospital beds while continuing to offer comprehensive care to chronic alcoholics.

Beginning in August 2003, hospital emergency rooms in San Francisco were able to transfer non–life-threatening inebriation cases to the McMillan Center, which will serve as a stabilization center. In September, the project moved into phase two, and paramedics were able to directly transport patients to the McMillan facility.

This project added 29 extra beds to the 140 emergency beds available in San Francisco. According to the Task Force, the project provides comprehensive care for chronic alcohol abusers, including individual case management, detoxification, and other health services, while freeing up bed space in the city's emergency rooms.

Chronic care settings

Challenging patients can be found in a variety of inpatient and outpatient settings. The description of the patient may vary, but strategies for dealing with difficult situations remain the same.

Mary Rau-Foster, RN, BS, ARM, JD, and president of Foster Seminars and Communications, is the author of *Dealing with Challenging Dialysis Patient Situations*. She has also written and produced a video-based training program and is a nationally known speaker on this topic.

Although initially written for clinicians who work with dialysis patients, many of these strategies are also effective with other patient populations in CCUs.

Foster offers the following guidance for dealing with challenging patients:

1. Provide rules and regulations to each patient when he or she first begins a relationship with your facility. Provide explanations and reasons for the rules and regulations and give the patient the opportunity to ask questions about them. Remind the patient of the rules when he or she fails to follow them.

2. Provide staff education and counseling. Providing the staff the opportunity to express their frustrations and concerns at the appropriate time and place is a necessary step in helping the patient. In addition, provide the employees with guidance and training in how to deal with and effectively communicate with patients who are being difficult.

3. Address concerns before they become problems. The Medicare Conditions of Participation requires that there be a grievance mechanism in place to allow the patients to express any concerns or problems that he or she may encounter. In addition, it is important to create an environment in which the patient does not fear retaliation for exercising this right.

4. Attempt to determine the nature, the contributing factors and possible solutions to the problems encountered with the challenging patient. This involves interviewing the patient to determine why he or she may be acting in a disruptive or difficult manner.

5. Clarify expectations with explanations. If there is an expectation that the patient needs to change certain behaviors or refrain from acting in a manner that is not conducive or appropriate for the environment, an explanation of what is expected of the patient is necessary. The focus should be on the behavior and not on the patient's personality.

6. Confront and counsel "one on one" with patient. Select an appropriate time and place where the counseling session could take place. The focus of the counseling session should be on the behavior(s) that needs to be changed.

7. Develop a plan of action with staff and patient input. The focus should be on how we might assist the patient in making the needed changes. Getting the patient's input regarding the cause of and solutions for the disruptive behavior may increase the likelihood of a successful outcome.

8. Try group counseling with the patient. It is important that certain members of the staff be present when the group counseling session takes place (medical director, administrator, nurse manager, social worker). The purpose and mechanics of the meeting should be planned out in advance. This meeting should focus on problem issues and what steps need to be taken to correct the problems. Care should be taken to create an environment conducive to problem identification and resolution, and not one of intimidation.

9. Document all steps taken with the patient and staff regarding the nature and context of the conflict. Be factual, objective, and specific in the documentation of any counseling sessions with the patient.

10. A contract that outlines what behavioral changes are necessary in order to continue the relationship may be an effective tool to use with some patients. This agreement should be specific and applicable to that patient and to his or her disruptive or difficult behaviors. It should not only address what is expected of the patient, but the agreement should also identify what the patient can expect from us, as healthcare providers.

11. Termination of the relationship with a patient should occur only as a last resort and when all other options have been exhausted. It is important to remember that a facility cannot terminate a relationship with a patient solely because the patient is not being compliant with his or her treatment prescription. However, the patient's nephrologist may terminate his or her relationship with the patient because of noncompliance. The patient's relationship with the facility would also terminate at the same time if there were no other physicians on staff who are willing to accept the patient as a client.

If the termination becomes necessary, the patient must be given adequate notice of the last date of treatment (such as 30 days) and must be provided with a list of other dialysis providers and physicians in the geographical area.

In conclusion, being a dialysis patient or the provider of care to the dialysis patient can be difficult. As health care professionals charged with the responsibility of providing life-saving treatments to persons whose lives have been disrupted by this illness, we must remember to be compassionate and understanding.

This requires stepping back mentally and emotionally and viewing the patients from a different angle. It includes reviewing our expectations of the patients and how they should respond to the stresses of their lives. It also begs that the following question be pondered: "What kind of dialysis patient would I be?"

Intensive care unit

A patient is admitted to the ICU and suddenly takes a turn for the worse. The patient's family, often still grappling with their family member's illness, has to change gears and begin contemplating end-of-life issues.

Improving satisfaction by helping families with end-of-life issues

Many times end-of-life issues have not been discussed by a patient's family, and the stress of the sudden illness, combined with guilt, loss, conflict over decision-maker duties, and varying opinions on care plans, can manifest itself in dissatisfaction with care.

Nurse managers can work with a patient's family to prevent miscommunication of important information, explain end-of-life issues, and offer education and reassurance.
Some effective strategies include:

- Ease the family's distress by describing differences between symptoms of pain and normal reductions in breathing and organ function.

- Arrange a care conference for a patient's family.

- Appoint a spokesperson at the hospital so that all of the family can talk to one person rather than different people answering the calls of family members. This ensures that consistent information is given to the family, and eliminates a situation in which four different family members call and get the same information communicated differently by four different people. This type of miscommunication, which was discussed in Chapter 2, is what family members mistake for staff "stonewalling." At the least, this type of miscommunication leads to dissatisfaction with staff; at the worst, it could mean costly litigation for your organization.

- Discuss aspects of the care plan such as nutrition and hydration with a patient's family. Families need to understand that a body racked with disease is shutting down and no longer requires the calories and fluids it once did. Explain the concept of "comfort care" to families.

- Encourage nurses to give the family complete information about the patient's medical condition, including pros and cons of treatment options, in order to help them make informed decisions. Assisting patients and their families in confronting and dealing with end-of-life issues is an important part of the nurse's role as a patient advocate.

- Many families don't understand that intravenous (IV) fluids do not lengthen the life of a person with a terminal illness, and they may feel guilty when an IV is shut off. It's imperative for staff to explain the patient's declining state and how their body can't absorb these fluids. Continuing an IV on a dying patient may lead to pulmonary edema, a condition that can make the last few hours of a patient's life more difficult for both the patient and the family, due to increased respiratory distress. This is usually not the way family members want to remember a loved one's last minutes.

- Emotional and spiritual end-of-life issues are important to patients and their families. Make referrals to the hospital chaplain, hospice, and support groups, and offer them the option of bereavement counseling after their loved one has passed on. Some families may be uncertain how to act around their dying family member, especially if he or she is in a coma. Nursing staff can help by letting family know they can still communicate with their loved one.

Barbara Long, president of E-Savvy Communications in Jefferson City, Mo has more than 20 years of experience working in health care public relations. Several years ago, her father was admitted to the ICU, and Long had the opportunity to view care in the ICU as a family member rather than as a public relations professional.

The experience of caring for her late father has motivated Barbara to encourage nursing staff to work in tandem with their hospital public relations department to promote better communication between staff and patient families.

Long notes that 90% of the problems her family faced when her father was hospitalized were communication-based, and she claims the communications breakdown she experienced is not an anomaly.

Our country offers good hospital care to patients, but aspects of this care are not communicated with patients and their families at the bedside.

Rather than having hospitals bury information about their patient representatives at the back of patient information packets, Long suggests that staff do the following:

- Take a proactive approach in letting patients and families know who to contact regarding questions and concerns and educate families on the role of a patient representative.

- Encourage staff to be proactive in asking patients and their families for feedback on their ICU and hospital stay. Patient satisfaction surveys are good tools, but there is only so much information that can be garnered from a set of questions. Long advocates having ICU staff informally ask patients and families on the spot about their care experiences that day.

Another way to gauge what families think of the care experience in the ICU is to periodically listen to family conversations in the waiting room. They will give you a good idea of family concerns and trends to address within your department. Take on the role of mystery shopper in your organization to determine the level of care and service that your patients are receiving.

Long also suggests that physicians and nurses use private rooms when they want to discuss a patient's condition or prognosis with family. All too often these conversations occur in a waiting room, which offers no privacy for family members.

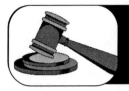

CASE STUDY: EXPLAINING PROTOCOLS IN SIMPLE TERMS

An elderly female patient had severe cognitive impairment and was suffering from end-stage Parkinson's disease. The physician asked the woman's daughter, "Is your mother coded DNR (do not resuscitate)?" The daughter said no, and the physician became exasperated, asking the daughter what quality of life she thought her mother had. This made the woman anxious, sending her into a confused panic.

The truth of the matter was no one had ever explained to the daughter the meaning of DNR. After the physician left, a nurse sat down with the daughter and reassured her that all her mother's needs would still be met; she would continue on an IV and receive appropriate care, but if her heart stopped, the staff would not administer cardiopulmonary resuscitation (CPR).

She explained that conducting CPR on someone as frail as her mother would result in broken ribs and horrible pain. Once the procedure was explained, the daughter thanked the nurse for taking the time to explain the protocol and signed the forms listing her mother as DNR. The daughter had been under the common misconception that DNR meant that all interventions would be discontinued.

Does your nursing staff use medical jargon when speaking to patients? Often, taking a few minutes to explain protocols can make a huge difference with patients and their families. Never assume that patients and their families are familiar with medical acronyms and hospital jargon.

Chapter 8

ESTABLISHING POLICIES AND PROTOCOLS

CHAPTER 8

Establishing Policies and Protocols

Dealing with issues associated with difficult patient populations and their families is a process fraught with the potential for misunderstandings and anger on the part of all involved. Considering the issues facing health care professionals discussed earlier, it becomes apparent that a comprehensive, consistent approach to how staff deals with patients and associated issues is needed.

Development of policies, procedures, and practice guidelines, although often tedious, allows for consistent application of an organizationally approved approach to a variety of issues. There is a differing opinion among hospital defense experts as to the types and numbers of policies needed, but most would agree that every organization needs some.

Patient complaints

The Centers for Medicare and Medicaid (CMS) requires, through their Conditions of Participation, a process by which patients or family members may file a grievance or complaint. There are additional requirements from the Joint Commission on Accreditation of Healthcare Organizations (JCAHO) and often your state's department of health.

In light of this, it becomes incumbent on all health care organizations receiving federal funds and/or reimbursement to comply with the CMS requirements. Components of this requirement should include a notification to patients of the process by which they can file a complaint, how those complaints will be addressed, and how the organization will respond.

In light of the requirements and the need to define an organizational response, both a policy and a mechanism to log those complaints should be developed. Policies should be comprehensive and reasonable. Do not fall into the trap that many organizations do, by developing an unreasonable and burdensome policy with which compliance may be an issue.

The requirement for the process is there, as are the components, but the manner in which it is implemented is up to the organization. Figure 8.1 is an example of a hospital-wide policy that defines and describes the process for dealing with patients' complaints or grievances.

| Figure 8.1 | ▬▬▬ **Patient Complaint/Grievance Policy** ▬▬▬ |

Purpose

To describe the process of informing patients of their right to make a complaint and the process of documenting, responding to, and tracking patient complaints for purposes of consistency, compliance, tracking, and trending for quality improvement opportunities.

Scope

Hospital wide

Policy

I. REGULATIONS:

The patient complaint process is developed in accordance with Department of Health (DOH), JCAHO, and Health Care Financing Administration (HCFA) Conditions of Participation Patient rights Guidelines.

II. PATIENT NOTIFICATION

A. Patients are notified of their right to make a complaint at the time they are admitted to service.

B. If the patient is admitted as an inpatient through the Admitting Department the Admitting Registrar provides the patient with a copy of the Patient Feedback Notice. Patients are also informed of their right to make a complaint on the Patient Rights sheet.

Figure 8.1 ████ **Patient Complaint/Grievance Policy (cont.)** ████

C. Patient Feedback Notices are posted at registration areas in the outpatient areas.

D. Patient rooms include information on the patient feedback process.

III. COMPLAINT DEFINITION

Overlake Hospital takes all patient complaints seriously. We recognize that complaints are associated with individual perspectives and the definition of a complaint is subjective based on that perspective. A situation is not defined as a complaint if a patient is asking for something or some action that can be easily resolved for him/her.

IV. REPORT PATIENT COMPLAINTS

A. Patients receiving care or services

1. Patients are encouraged to notify their nurse or caregiver immediately if they have a complaint while they are receiving care or services.

2. If the patient is uncomfortable discussing the issue with his/her nurse or caregiver, or if the patient feels the issue has not been resolved to his/her satisfaction, the patient may choose to speak with the Charge Nurse or Department manager, or the patient may contact the Patient Action Line.

B. Discharged patients or patients not currently receiving care

Patient complaints that enter the system after the patient has been discharged or is not currently receiving care may enter the system in a variety of ways. It is the responsibility of the staff member who is notified of the patient complaint to attempt to resolve the issue if it is within their scope to do so. Issues that cannot be easily resolved for the patient or outside of the area of the person receiving the complaint are forwarded to the Patient Action Line for follow-up.

1. Patient complaints related to quality of care or premature discharge concerns may be shared with the Peer Review Organization of Washington.

Figure 8.1 ■■■■■■■ **Patient Complaint/Grievance Policy (cont.)** ■■■■■■■

V. PATIENT ACTION LINE

The Patient Action Line is available to patients and family members 24 hours a day, 7 days a week.

Calls and information received on the Patient Action Line are reviewed by the hospital representative and forwarded to the appropriate Clinical or Department Manager for additional follow-up and problem solving if needed.

Calls and information received on the Patient Action Line that meet the definition of Patient Complaint, as defined in Section III above, are entered into the Patient Complaint database for tracking and trending purposes.

VI. COMPLAINT RESEARCH/DETERMINATION OF ACTION

A. The Clinical or Department Manager or Director is primarily responsible for follow-up on patient complaint issues related to his/her department. Research may include follow up with staff, the Risk Manager, and other areas as needed.

B. Complaints involving the Medical Staff are forwarded to the Director of medical Staff Services.

C. In some cases, patient complaints may be reviewed by the appropriate Committee to determine recommendations for action and follow-up. Examples of Committees that may be involved in the review process include:

1. Quality Improvement Committee

2. Professional Advisory Committees

D. It is the responsibility of the Clinical or Department Manager or Director to ensure follow-up and action steps taken for resolution are added to the Patient Complaint database.

VII. RESPONSE TO PATIENT

It is the responsibility of the Clinical or Department Manager or Director, or other hospital representative, if defined otherwise during the complaint research process, to respond to the patient in writing within 10 business days from the time the complaint was received. Information contained in the letter will include:

| Figure 8.1 | **Patient Complaint/Grievance Policy (cont.)** |

- Name of contact person

- Steps taken to research the complaint

- Results/action steps that will be taken

- Date of completion

If resolution has not yet occurred, the letter will specify an estimated date for resolution and at that time, an additional letter will be sent to the patient.

VIII. PATIENT COMPLAINT SUMMARIES

  Patient complaint report summaries are periodically reviewed with the Quality

  Improvement Committee and Quality, Compliance, and Cost Effectiveness

  Committee of the Board.

Source: Overlake Hospital Medical Center

A policy should also define and outline instances of patient abuse, neglect, and unprofessional/ unethical conduct on the part of an employee. Figure 8.2 is a sample policy taken from a rehabilitation department that accomplishes this well.

Patients' rights and responsibilities

Clear, consistent communication will reduce complaints and the potential for misunderstanding. Clearly outlining the patient's rights and responsibilities establishes a framework on which the communication process can be built.

It is recommended that health care facilities not only provide a patient's rights document but also include in it his or her responsibilities. If in fact we believe that there is a partnership with the patient, we should establish what his or her role is (see Figure 8.3). By doing this, you are communicating that respect and responsibility between your staff and your patients are to be mutual.

| Figure 8.2 | **Abuse, Neglect, Conduct, Complaints Policy** |

Purpose	The Rehabilitation Center Policies and Procedures Manual is designed to provide a ready reference file to current unit operational and practice guidelines and is applicable to all unit personnel and practice guidelines; and to assure that all persons in the Rehabilitation Center are treated with dignity and respect.
Audience	All members of the Rehabilitation Center Program.
Policy	All persons served by the Rehabilitation Center shall be treated with dignity and respect. It is the responsibility of the Rehabilitation Center to assure that all employees will refrain from behaviors that are unprofessional, unethical, illegal, abusive or neglectful. It is also the policy that all employees can identify any occurrence of abuse, neglect, unprofessional and unethical conduct and take appropriate action. This policy also affords the patient an opportunity to have his or her grievance investigated and responded to in a timely manner.
Inservice Education	The Rehabilitation Center will provide a minimum of 8 hours of inservice education annually to all employees to assist them in identifying patient abuse or neglect and illegal, unprofessional, or unethical conduct by or in the facility. The inservice will also provide each employee with the grievance procedure policy as it applies to all patients in the adult rehabilitation unit.
Component of Service	The inservice training program shall contain: 1. Instruction designed to improve patient care and prevent abuse, neglect, and unethical conduct from occurring. 2. Instruction on specific types of patient abuse and neglect and how to identify when abuse or neglect is occurring or has occurred.

Figure 8.2 █████████ **Abuse, Neglect, Conduct, Complaints Policy (cont.)** ████████

3. Instruction on specific types of illegal, unprofessional and unethical conduct, and how to identify when illegal, unprofessional, and unethical conduct is occurring or has occurred.

4. Instruction on the requirements and procedures for reporting any incidence of patient abuse and neglect or unethical, illegal, or unprofessional conduct together with the instructions on the applicable penalties for not reporting an occurrence.

5. Detailed information on the legal protection afforded to employees and associated health care professionals who report patient abuse and neglect and illegal, unprofessional, and unethical conduct.

Documentation of Inservices	The Rehabilitation Center shall keep on record documentation of completion of this required training.

1. Documentation shall contain a description of the training content, the date or dates on which the training was received, and the number of hours attended on each date.

2. Documentation must be signed and dated by the employee and the instructor or supervisor.

3. Documentation must be retained for 10 years.

Patient Grievance Procedure	1. Patients or patients' family members registering a complaint with any Rehabilitation Center personnel will have

Figure 8.2 ▬ **Abuse, Neglect, Conduct, Complaints Policy (cont.)** ▬

their complaint identified as a grievance. The personnel member is required to report the grievance to the patients' program manager or nurse manager. The patient will be informed of the Rehabilitation Center Grievance Procedure and the patient or patients' family member may choose to follow the grievance procedure or contact UTMB Patient Services at 772-4772. The grievance will be documented in the patient grievance data base by the program manager and an investigation will begin within a 24-hour period of time once reported to the program or nurse manager. If the grievance involves abuse or neglect, the Rehabilitation Center personnel receiving the complaint has the additional responsibility of reporting it to the Administrative Director.

2. If the resolution offered to the patient or patients' family member (the party that initiated the grievance) agrees that the complaint is resolved, the matter ends at the informal level. Each member, party to the grievance, is notified. The resolution is documented in the patient grievance data base, which identifies that the issue was resolved and documents the resolution that occurred.

3. If it cannot be resolved at this level, the patient of patients' family member may choose to initiate a formal grievance. This step is coordinated by the program manager or nurse manager.

4. An Ad-Hoc Committee appointed and chaired by the Administrative Director or her designee will meet to review

the grievance within a 72-hour period of initiation of the formal grievance. The committee should be composed of disinterested parties from within the Adult Rehab Unit, one member for Patient Relations, and no less than one additional member from UTMB personnel outside the unit and/or the direct supervisor(s) of the service(s) in question. All involved parties must submit a written summation and may be called to the meeting for additional information.

5. The committee will make a recommendation for resolution or provide a status report within a 24-hour period of the meeting. The patient will be informed of the outcome of the grievance committee and all parties involved will receive written notification of the outcome, along with the medical director. The resolution will be signed (agree or disagree) by all direct parties and forwarded to the UTMB Clinical Risk Manager coordinator and documented in the patient grievance data base.

6. The patient may still contact patient services at 772-4772 if they are not fully satisfied with the sanctions of the grievance committee.

7. In all cases, if the grievance involves neglect, abuse, or illegal or unprofessional behavior the patient maintains the right to contact the Texas Department of Health Information Complaint Line at 1-800-228-1570 or the Texas Department of Protective and Regulator Services at 1-800-252-5400.

Source: The University of Texas Medical Branch

| Figure 8.3 | Patients' Rights and Responsibilities |

You have the RIGHT to:

- Considerate, respectful care and treatment without regard to race, creed, sex, national origin or source of payment.

- Be informed of your health status and involved in your care planning and decisions and in resolving dilemmas about care decisions that may occur.

- Include participation of your family or representatives in care decisions when appropriate.

- Have your spiritual needs met through chaplains, visiting clergy or qualified volunteers.

- Make a complaint. This includes the right to contact the Department of health at 1-900-633-6838 if you have concerns that have not been resolved to [y]our satisfaction by the hospital.

- Formulate advance directives, orders to withhold resuscitate services and/or forgo or withdraw life-sustaining treatment and have hospital staff comply with the directives.

- Have family or your representative or physician notified promptly of any admission to the hospital.

- Be free from any form of restraints (physical or chemical) when they are used as a form of coercion, discipline, convenience or retaliation.

- Appropriate assessment and management of pain.

- Accept or refuse the care and treatment offered.

- Accept or refuse to participate in research studies.

- Privacy when being interviewed, examined, and treated.

- Confidentiality of health care information and to expect that all information shared will be done so according to federal and state laws and regulations.

- Review all or any part of your medical record and, upon request, receive and copy of all or any part of your medical record, and to request an amendment or correction in your medical record. Expect reasonable safety insofar as hospital practices and environment are concerned and to access protective services when considered necessary for your personal safety.

Figure 8.3 ██████████ **Patient's Rights and Responsibilities (cont.)** ██████

- Be free from all forms of abuse or harassment.
- Have access to people outside of the hospital (this includes visitors and/or verbal and written communication).
- Refuse to see anyone not officially connected with the hospital or your care.
- Have the services of an interpreter (when available) and/or access to telecommunication devices for the deaf if you do not speak or understand the language of the community.
- Be transferred to another facility only after you have received a complete explanation of the need for such a transfer.
- Receive information about continuing health care requirements following your discharge.
- Know who is responsible for authorizing and performing any procedures or treatment.
- Receive an itemized and detailed explanation of your hospital bill when requested.

You have the Responsibility to:

- Provide, to the best of your ability, accurate and complete details about your past illnesses, hospitalizations, medications and present conditions.
- Tell your doctor about a change in your condition or if problems arise.
- Tell your doctor or nurse if you do not understand your treatment or what you are expected to do.
- Pay your bill promptly or to tell the hospital if you are unable to pay your bill.
- Notify the hospital about who is responsible for the bill if you are not paying.

Source: Overlake Hospital Medical Center

Complex case management and discharge planning

Screening patients for assignment of the level of case management and discharge planning they will need preserves resources and allows for an opportunity early in a patient's stay to begin the process of discharge planning for the complex patient.

Figure 8.4 is a sample policy for identifying patients who may be candidates for complex case management needs. The policy outlines risk factors that indicate patients may require additional resources. Social workers can use this criteria to screen patients for case managers.

Figure 8.4 ■ **High-Risk Criteria: Intensive Case Management & Complex Discharge** ■

Policy: All social workers will be aware of risk factors that may require patients to have intensive case management and complex discharge planning needs while hospitalized.

1. Social workers will screen for the following factors that may include but are not limited to:

   A. Patients admitted from Nursing Homes
   B. Patients admitted from Retirement Homes, Assisted Living Facilities, or Adult Family Homes
   C. Patients already receiving Home health services at the time of Hospital admission
   D. Patients 65 years old and have additional risk factors
   E. Geriatric patients who are unkempt or poorly nourished on admission
   F. Patients with a history of dementia, cognitive impairment, or psychiatric illness that impacts understanding and ability to comply with treatment
   G. Patients who will require complex wound care of new ostomy care after discharge
   H. Patients admitted with trauma sustained injuries
   I. Patients on new or chronic renal dialysis
   J. Homeless adults
   K. Patients with limited social support that might benefit from a screening for Senior Care referral
   L. Patients with a history of Dementia

Figure 8.4 **High-Risk Criteria (cont.)**

M. Patients with multiple physician consultations

N. Patients with length of stay greater than 5 days

O. All patients of the Physical Medicine and Rehabilitation Service

P. Ventilator dependent patients

Q. All medically admitted patients with overdoses

R. Patients with multiple re-admissions

S. Patients with behavioral issues that impact their hospital care, such as abusive behavior toward staff

T. Treatment withdrawal, end of life decision making

U. Patients requiring multi-disciplinary conferencing/planning

V. Patients with active Adult or Child Protective Services involvement (APS/CPS)

W. Patients with alcohol or other substance abuse

X. Patients with poor understanding and comprehension regarding treatment compliance

Y. Patients requiring assistance with dressing change

Z. Patients with little or no family support

2. Awareness and implementation if:

A. Domestic violence Protocol is met

B. Duty to report abuse, suspected abuse or neglect of a child, vulnerable adult, or developmentally disabled person

3. Participation with other providers in assessment of the Mother/Baby Unit will include:

A. Participation in Pathways for normal vaginal and C-section as indicated by criteria

B. Awareness and implementation of the following:
   1. Social Work intervention and discharge planning on Perinatal Unit
   2. Adoption protocol
   3. Protocol for fetal demise
   4. Scheduled C-section clinical pathway
   5. Normal vaginal delivery clinical pathway

Figure 8.4 ■■■■■■■■■■■ **High-Risk Criteria (cont.)** ■■■■■■■■■

4. Participation with other providers in assessment for the psychiatric unit will include:

  A. Inpatient psychiatric protocols for Social Work intervention and discharge planning
  B. Dual diagnosis Clinical Pathway
  C. Axis II clinical Pathway
  D. Adolescent patients standard of care

Source: Overlake Hospital Medical Center

It also would be beneficial to clearly establish the nurse's role in discharge planning (see Figure 8.5). A comprehensive and consistent approach to this process for staff can potentially decrease the likelihood of a patient being noncompliant and not following the suggested treatment plan.

Admission status

A lack of understanding on the part of staff, physicians, patients, and families of admission status is almost guaranteed. This complex process most commonly occurs in the elderly population, although not exclusively. A clear explanation of the decision making process provides the greatest likelihood of compliance with CMS requirements and, more importantly, a basis for explaining to patients and families why a particular status has been assigned.

As we discussed in Chapter 1, confusion over status and its effect on discharge planning and reimbursement (i.e., who will cary the burden of the cost of services) often leads to a difficult situation with a patient or his or her family. The importance of developing a policy to ensure consistency in your organization's decision making process is clearly evident.

Figure 8.5
Nurse's Role in Discharge Planning

PURPOSE
To outline guidelines for the nurse to provide the patient and/or family with knowledge, skills, and resources required to meet the patient's ongoing health care needs after discharge.

STEPS → KEY POINTS

1. Assessment of patient's discharge needs will be initiated and documented at the time of the patient's admission by the RN. (See Admission of Patient policy, JCAHO Requirement.)

2. The following criteria are used to screen patients at the time of admission for discharge planning by Social Work Services. A referral will be made to Social Services Worker if any of the following conditions exists.

- History of drug/alcohol abuse

- Frail elderly

- Hx repeat admits

- Needs assistance at home after discharge to care for self or family

- Catastrophic illness or injury

- Hx or recent onset of psychiatric illness

- Behavioral management issue

- Need for crisis intervention

- Admitted from nursing home, retirement center, or adult family home

- Admitted while being followed by home health agency

- Concerns related to patient's home situation

- Fall Risk Assessment score >4

- Any other health care/patient/family concerns

3. Multidisciplinary discharge preparation will include:
- Safe and effective medication use.
- Safe and effective use of any medical equipment.

| Figure 8.5 | ■■■■■■ **Nurse's Role in Discharge Planning (cont.)** ■■■■■■ |

- Instruction of potential drug-food interactions and counseling on nutrition intervention and/or modified diets.

- Instruction in rehabilitation techniques to facilitate adaptation to and/or functional independence in the environment.

- Access to available community resources.

- When and how to obtain further treatment.

DOCUMENTATION

1. At the time of discharge, the RN/LPN will complete the Discharge Record. (See Documentation: Discharge Record policy.)

2. The RN and other disciplinarians will document discharge preparation and teaching on the patient's record (This may include and is not limited to Patient Teaching Record, 24-hour Patient Care Flow Sheet, Kardex Care Plan, Clinical Pathway, Care Conference, Progress Notes or unit/department specific documentation forms.

Source: Overlake Hospital Medical Center

Equally important and equally sensitive is a clear policy or guideline by which placement in a long-term care facility is decided (see Figure 8.6).

Long-term placement

As discussed in Chapter 2, funding for long-term care is always a controversial matter, as is the realization that a parent or spouse may need to be transferred to a facility on discharge from the hospital. This is a decision fraught with emotion for everyone involved. A policy related to placement makes everyone's job a little easier.

Figure 8.6 is a sample policy that outlines the decision-making process for patients who are possible candidates for placement in a long-term care facility.

| Figure 8.6 | **Guidelines for Nursing Home Placement** |

I. Determining When a Patient Needs Nursing Home Placement

A. Assessment Criteria

  1. MD, Nursing referral or Social Work Coordinator high risk screening, based upon patient's History and Physical or nursing admission history.

  2. Patient/family request based upon perceived care needs.

  3. Patients evaluated by the Rehabilitation Medicine Services as meeting the criteria for sub-acute rehabilitation.

  4. Patients who have new mobility limitations/needs. When a change in patients condition exceeds what their usual caregiver can provide and have new mobility limitations/needs.

  5. Patients who need short term rehabilitation (OT, PT, ST) as a result of their acute hospitalization. Following subacute rehab, patients may return home, or may go on to long-term custodial care.

  6. Patients on clinical pathways that are not progressing as expected on the pathway, and appear not ready to return directly home to recover.

  7. Patient's requiring comfort/terminal care, and are not imminently terminal.

B. Implementation of a Nursing Home Placement

  1. Review the medical record and consult other team members in regard to a patient's care needs.

| Figure 8.6 | ▇▇▇▇▇ **Guidelines for Nursing Home Placement (cont.)** ▇▇▇▇▇ |

2. Interview patient, and/or family to assess their understanding and need for placement. Provide information, education as needed.

3. Review financial reimbursement sources available in light of patient's medical condition and care needs (Medicare, Medicaid, Labor and industry, private health care insurance, third party insurance, long-term care insurance, and private pay).

4. Offer options available on skilled nursing facilities to patient, and/or family, considering:
   • Physical location
   • Reimbursement source and requirements (preferred providers with insurance)
   • Bed availability (this may require first, second and third choices)
   • Patient care needs

5. Either the Social Work Coordinator of family can check on bed availability. Recommend that the family visit facilities before making their selection.

6. When a facility is selected, contact their Admissions Coordinator and fax the following information:
   • Patient's fact sheet
   • Anticipated discharge date
   • Name of insurance case manager if known
   • Admission History and Physical
   • Medication sheets (MAR)
   • One of two days of nursing notes
   • Graphics sheet (documents IV fluid administration)
   • PT/OT/ST progress notes and summary as appropriate
   • Transfer Form (if already completed by MD)
   • Discharge Summary (if already completed by MD)

Figure 8.6 ███████ **Guidelines for Nursing Home Placement (cont.)** ███████

7. Once the MD has determined the patient's discharge date, transportation will be coordinated by the Social Work Coordinator/HUC/Family, in conjunction with recommendations by the MD, Nursing, and PT. The unit HUC will be notified of patient's method of transportation. The Patient and family will be advised of transportation alternatives-car/cabulance/ambulance. Medical necessity of ambulance transport and insurance pre-authorization of ambulance of cabulance (if part of patient's insurance benefits) will also be reviewed by the patient and/or family. The Social Work Coordinator will document patient or family agreement to private paying cabulance or ambulance transportation in the patient's chart.

8. Each nursing unit designee will compile the following information packet to accompany the patient to the skilled nursing facility:
   • Completed Transfer Form
   • Recent lab work, x-rays, CT's, report of operation
   • Admission History and Physical
   • Discharge Summary
   • OBRA-PASSARR form completed by the Social Work Coordinator
   • Copy of Advanced Directives

II. Special Considerations in Regard to Insurance Coverage of Skilled Nursing Facility Care

A. Patient and Family Education

1. Medicare and insurance definition of "skilled" versus "custodial" levels of care. Medicare and some private insurance plans do not reimburse for custodial level care.

2. Review the basics of how a nursing facility may determine how long a patient may be funded (how a patient may be assessed as meeting skilled criteria by Medicare or other insurance companies.)

Figure 8.6 ■ **Guidelines for Nursing Home Placement (cont.)** ■

3. Encourage that family review the patient's long-term care insurance polity, and its potential applicability in patient's current situation.

4. Discuss with patient and family how the Medicare and managed care sponsored patient may be located in an area separate from long term care residents.

III. OBRA-PASSARR Requirements

A. Social Work Coordinator completes OBRA-PASSARR form prior to patient's transfer to a skilled nursing facility. This requirement applies only to Medicaid certified nursing facilities, regardless if Medicare, Medicaid, other insurance or private pay will fund patient's stay.

B. If there is a "Yes" response to any of the questions in Section A or B, the patient must be screened for one of two steps. The first is to evaluate for the use of the "PASSARR Exemption Verification" form. This form is applicable when an MD states that the patient will be transferred directly from an acute care hospital to a SNF for a condition that the patient was hospitalized and treated, for less than 30 days of skilled nursing care. The patient's attending MD completes and signs the form. The second step requires that the referral must be faxed to DSHS Aging and Adult Services.

C. A PASSARR (OBRA) form must be completed on all patients entering a Medicaid certified nursing home, regardless of whether they will initially be funded by Medicare, Medicaid or the patient will private pay.

D. Psychiatric consultation by the Overlake Hospital consulting psychiatrist can be useful in assessing whether patients have a "serious mental illness" if the MD and the Case Manager are unsure or if the patient has emotional or behavioral problems.

| Figure 8.6 | ▬▬▬▬▬ **Guidelines for Nursing Home Placement (cont.)** ▬▬▬▬ |

IV. Special Consideration For Medicaid Patients

    A. Patients without insurance to fund nursing home placement or whose insurance only pays for "skilled" care, and the patient has "custodial" needs.

        1. If the patient appears to meet the income and asset guidelines, and is not already on Medicaid, refer to the Patient/family to the DSHS Aging and Aging and Adult Services, Alternate Care Unit.

        2. Briefly review with the patient/family, Medicaid financial process. Have the patient/family advise DSHS if there is a "bed waiting", which may facilitate the application turnaround time. Some skilled nursing facilities will also accept a patient as "Medicaid pending" the application has been submitted and pending approval. Also have the patient/family convey this information to DSHS if applicable.

Source: Overlake Hospital Medical Center

Care conferences

Complex decisions involving multiple parties may be required to resolve issues related to initial, ongoing, follow-up, and even end-of-life care. It is beneficial, in times where there are numerous parties involved to facilitate a care conference. Ground rules and a process outline increases the ease with which staff will initiate and participate in such meetings (see Figure 8.7).

Figure 8.7
Care Conference Policy

DEFINITION

Care Conference: A multi-disciplinary health-care team collaboration for the assessment, development and delivery of a patient care plan.

SUPPORTIVE INFORMATION

Any health care professional can initiate a Care Conference.

The multidisciplinary health care team will collaborate with the patient/family/significant other (S.O.) to identify a patient's specific care needs and interventions needed.

The RN will integrate, plan and monitor outcomes to ensure that the needs of each patient are met in a timely manner. A multidisciplinary approach will be used.

Goals of the Care Conference:

- Provide consistent care from shift to shift.
- Anticipate patient needs and provide appropriate patient care.
- Eliminate duplication of services.
- Provide collaboration of care that will best benefit the patient/family/significant other (S.O.).
- Identify clinical interventions that are effective
- Address discharge issues
- Key Point → The Kardex/Care Plan will continue to be used for care needs/interventions that are not on the Care Conference form.

STEPS → KEY POINTS

1. Identify the need for a Care Conference and invite the multidisciplinary health care team.

2. A Care Conference form will be used to document the information. This is a permanent part of the patient's record.

| Figure 8.7 | Care Conference Policy (cont.) |

3. Place the Care Conference form (Kardex/Care Plan and Clinical Pathways) in the patient's chart, in front of the patient's 24-hour Patient Care Flow Sheet or per unit-specific protocol.

4. Complete the appropriate sections of the Care Conference form.

5. The RN or other health care team member will indicate the care needs or medical/nursing issue to be addressed.

6. The RN or other health care team member will document date of the Care Conference on the Kardex/Care Plan.

7. To schedule a Care Conference, the Health Unit Coordinator (HUC) or person entering orders, will enter in the computer the date and time the Care Conference will be held. Enter order as for any other order entry.
   a. On the Order Entry screen under Category, enter CCR (all caps), Care Coordinator Rounds.

   b. Under Procedure, Look Up (F9) to see the List of Consults:
      • CNS (send an email or make a phone call; do not check)
      • Infection Control Nurse
      • Nutritional Services
      • Occupational Therapist
      • Pharmacist
      • Psych Department Members
      • Physical Therapist
      • Respiratory Therapist
      • Speech Therapist
      • Social Worker
      • Chaplain

Figure 8.7

Care Conference Policy (cont.)

c. Check the consultants (health team members) to attend. Note the instructions at the bottom of the screen: Use the right Ctrl Key to check. Us the down and up arrows to scroll.

d. OK (F12) will take you back to the Order screen.

8. If any other disciplines such as the receiving nursing unit charge nurse/staff nurse, CNS, physician, etc., are required to attend the Care Conference, notify them by a computer message or phone call.

9. The date of the Care Conference will be indicated on the patient's Kardex/Care Plan in the appropriate section under Discharge Prep & Education by the patient's nurse assisting in the Care Conference or the HUC.

10. If time allows, the day prior to the Care Conference a memo will be posted by the patient's nurse assisting in the Care Conference or the HUC identifying the date and time of the Care Conference.

11. The patient's nurse will inform the Charge Nurse of the date and time of the conference. The Charge Nurse will make any staffing or assignment adjustments to allow for the Care Conference patient's RN to attend the Care Conference.

12. The Care Conference form will be supplemented to the care planning on the Kardex/Care Plan and will not replace the Kardex/Care Plan.

13. Any RN or LPN may revise the plan identified in a Care Conference. This can be done by:
- Initiating another Care Conference.
- Updating the current Care Conference by dating and signing (under the original date) and starting or stopping an intervention by dating and initiating in the Start & Stop section of the Care Conference form.
- If a new intervention is needed, add the intervention to the generic or unit-based Kardex/Care Plan.

14. See Documentation: Kardex/Care Plan policy.

Source: Overlake Hospital Medical Center

Interpretation services

It is a facility's legal and moral obligation to provide care to the immigrant population. At a minimum, facilities should establish an effective method for providing interpretive services. Any policy related to provision of this service should define what a qualified interpreter is and how to go about obtaining one. If there are variables in how the policy should be applied, those too should be clearly identified (see Figure 8.8).

Substance abusers

Many of the issues regarding plans of care, case management, care conferences, and discharge planning apply to patients who present in the emergency department (ED) and are identified as substance abusers. This population requires intense case management to reduce the frequency of their visits to acute care facilities by increasing their outpatient compliance.

Mechanisms for early identification of substance abuse should be incorporated into assessments, and policies regarding the management of intoxicated patients should be clear. Like most of the populations discussed in this book, intoxicated patients are difficult to deal with, especially when that is their sole reason for being in an ED. However, health care facilities have a duty to ensure that before discharge, they are free of other potentially harmful medical problems and are safe for discharge.

Since these patients are frequently in the facilities after regular business hours, it is important to provide staff with guidance on how to manage them. Figure 8.9 is a sample procedure for dealing with these potentially difficult patients.

Figure 8.8	**Interpretive Services-for Non-English Speaking Patients**

PURPOSE

To provide guidelines to ensure that all non-English speaking Overlake Hospital Medical Center patients have access to effective, accurate and impartial interpretive services.

SUPPORTIVE INFORMATION

It is the policy of Overlake Hospital Medical Center to meet the health care needs of our non-English speaking patients. Overlake Hospital Medical Center will provide access to qualified foreign language interpretive services for all non-English speaking patients through specific contracted interpretive services agencies at no cost to the patient. Upon the request of the physician, patient or hospital staff, services may be accessed in the following circumstances (including but not limited to): provide emergency assessment and services; obtain informed consent; provide discharge instruction; provide information regarding surgical and diagnostic procedures; and to translate any and all information either orally or in writing, if related to the above and/or patient's condition, diagnostic testing or course of treatment.

DEFINITIONS

Qualified interpreter: A sign/oral interpreter who has demonstrated a high level of expressive and receptive skills and thorough knowledge of the Code of Ethics on Interpreting, or a person who speaks English and another language fluently enough to accurately and effectively communicate, including an understanding of the nonverbal and cultural patterns of the language.

Specific Contracted Agencies: Agencies with which Overlake Hospital Medical Center has entered into a specific contract to provide interpretive services.

STEPS KEY → POINTS

Obtaining Interpretive Services

1. Hospital personnel should obtain the following information prior to requesting interpretive services:
   - Emergent or non-emergent request
   - Correct language and/or dialect
   - Department name, phone number and name of person making request

Figure 8.8	**Interpretive Services Policy (cont.)**

- Date, time and length of time required for the appointment
- Medicaid PIC or case number (see Medicaid Outpatients/ER Patients)
- Additional information as appropriate, i.e. gender preference

2. Once the need for interpretive services is determined, it will be the responsibility of the charge nurse to make the request for services and to place the "Services Documentation" form in the patient's chart.

3. To request services for non-English speaking patients during business hours, call the Social Services Program Assistant at (omit). Requests for pre-scheduled, non-emergent verbal language services should be made at least 24 hours in advance.

4. After normal business hours, the nurse must notify the Shift Administrator. The Shift Administrator will assist by calling the appropriate service.

5. If the request for services is for a pre-scheduled surgery patient, Social Services will initiate the "Services Documentation" form and forward it to the appropriate unit to be placed in the patient's chart.

6. If the number of hours of services required by the patient exceeds two (2) hours, the charge nurse must notify and obtain the approval of the Social Worker Supervisor or the Director of Social Workers prior to completing the form during business hours.

7. Patients who decline the use of the qualified services provided by Overlake Hospital Medical Center may rely on family or friends when:

- Hospital personnel determine that the patient fully understands the availability of these services.
- The patient fully understands that there is no additional cost associated with interpretive services.
- The patient understands that despite the current refusal, he/she may request and will be provided with such services at any time during hospitalization.

| Figure 8.8 | Interpretive Services Policy (cont.) |

Cancellation of Services

If the need arises to cancel or change an appointment, please call Social Services Program Assistant at (omit). After normal business hours, please call the Shift Administrator. Document the reason for the cancellation or change in the patient's medical record.

DOCUMENTATION

1. Medical Record: The following information will be documented in the patient's medical record on the "Interpretive Services" form.
   - Language of the patient and need for interpretive services
   - Date and time the request was made
   - Reason interpreter needed (see codes)
   - Who will be interpreting (family, friend, staff agency)
   - Name of interpreter used
   - Date and time the interpreter was provided

2. Encounter Form: The interpreter must present this form to be completed and signed by the charge nurse. The signed form will be forwarded to Social Services by the services agency.

Source: Overlake Hospital Medical Center

| Figure 8.9 | ▆▆▆ | **Substance Abuse Evaluation in the Emergency Department** | ▆▆▆ |

Patients present to the Emergency Department with alcohol, or other substance abuse problems. Patients may present intoxicate, in acute withdrawal, or in no apparent distress, requesting assistance in locating treatment resources. Substance abuse may be the primary presenting problem, or may be concurrent with a psychiatric problem, or a medical problem.

First, assess the safety of the patient. If the patient has made suicidal statements, or actions, his/her alcohol level must be 100 or less to assess suicidal risk. If a patient has a concurrent psychiatric problem requiring psychiatric admission, or referral to CDMHP's the patient's alcohol level must be 100 or less before a treatment contract is signed, or before CDMHP referral is made. Historical information may be gathered while the patient is intoxicated, depending upon the cooperativeness level of the patient. An intoxicated patient presenting as a danger to him/herself or others may be restrained if necessary. The Emergency Department physician must order restraints. When the patient's blood alcohol level is below 100, complete the psych evaluation form and make appropriate disposition plan.

Patients presenting without a concurrent psychiatric problem, or suicidal risk, may be assessed while intoxicated, if necessary. Assessment should include:

1. Current substance use- types, frequency, amounts, and reason for Emergency
   Department visit.
2. History of substance abuse use-onset, types, methods used, past treatment, impatient
   or outpatient, and length of sobriety after treatment.
3. Current motivation for treatment-outpatient versus inpatient, financial resources.

Patients presenting in withdrawal or remission should be assessed as above, and appropriate disposition plan made.

The Emergency Department physician is the person to determine medical incapacity secondary to substance intoxication or withdrawal, and can authorize the use of restraints in such situation, even if the patient is not suicidal. Generally, a person being discharged with an alcohol level over 100 will need a responsible adult, willing to monitor the patient during the remainder of his/her intoxication.

Source: Overlake Hospital Medical Center

Chapter 9

DOCUMENTING THE DIFFICULT PATIENT EXPERIENCE

CHAPTER 9

Documenting the Difficult Patient Experience

Nurses today need to be aware of the increasing number of lawsuits filed by patients dissatisfied with their care. This fact, coupled with how the country's nursing shortage is forcing nurses to take on more responsibility and accountability for patients in the acute care setting, means nurses are increasing their chances of being named in a lawsuit.

The primary reason for documenting care—difficult patients or otherwise—is to provide subsequent health care providers with information regarding the previous episode of care. This may be the previous shift, the previous 24 hours, or in some instances, the previous office visit or hospitalization.

It is a health care provider's responsibility to chart what has occurred during his or her shift and, just as important, to read what has occurred on the previous shifts. This has become increasingly important, as staffing patterns may not always give the same nurse the same assignment day after day.

It is also important to keep in mind the old nursing adage, "If it wasn't charted, it didn't happen," and realize that accurate documentation plays a crucial defense if a patient decides to file a lawsuit. If your nurses maintain good documentation at all times, it will reduce liability in a number of ways.

When nurse managers discuss proper charting protocols, they should make their staff aware of the cases attorneys can make by dissecting sloppy, incomplete documentation. Staff need to understand that in addition to being clear, good documentation should illustrate that a difficult patient was informed of the care you provided and the role he or she played in that care.

Documenting difficult situations

Charting difficult patient situations or confrontations that may lead to possible legal ramifications demands good judgment. Here are some guidelines to follow that will protect nurses and their employers from litigation troubles:

Don't refer to staffing problems

If a nurse feels that inadequate staffing affected a patient's care, he or she should follow the hospital's policy for reporting the problem. Appropriate actions include writing a confidential memo, completing an incident report, or notifying the unit supervisor and making a personal note (not in the chart) that he or she called the situation to the attention of their nurse manager.

Avoid wording that implies errors were made

When charting, nurses should avoid words that imply that errors have been made. Words such as "accidentally" or "unintentionally" can easily be interpreted as admissions of errors. If an order is not carried out correctly, nurses should indicate in the chart what happened and what actions were taken.

Include behaviors that interfere with treatment

Nurses must document all patient behaviors that interfere with medical treatment, and they need to include information in the chart that shows that patients have been notified of the possible consequences of their actions. For example, document that you explained to the patient that if he or she refuses to use a walker for assistance, the likelihood of a fall and subsequent injuries increases.

Exclude your opinions

The chart is a place for facts, not the opinions of nursing staff. If a nurse is unhappy with his or her patient, the physician, or the facility, the chart is not the place to "vent." Charting criticism make nurses appear less credible. If a nurse has concerns about staffing issues or the patient's care plan, they should be addressed through the proper channels, not in a patient's chart.

Document what is said

It is just as critical to document what a patient says to you as it is to document his or her condition.

Does a patient tell you that he or she does not understand the treatment plan?

Have patients told you they don't want to be a burden to their families?

Are they concerned about the resources they might need after being discharged

from the hospital?

It is important for nurses to document patient conversations like these, which might help defuse future problems and will be useful in the case management of this type of patient.

Record unauthorized possessions

Nurses should document any unusual or unauthorized items that the patient possesses. Such items may include alcoholic beverages, tobacco, heating pads, medications brought from home, or devices that should be checked by the biomedical department before use. Describe each item in a narrative note and what action you took to dispose of the item.

Note when the patient disregards the physician's advice

If a patient chooses to be discharged against the advice of his or her physician, nurses need to document the patient's request to leave in the patient's own words and how the consequences of his or her actions were fully explained. This is a way to ensure you have kept the patient involved and informed in his or her own care.

Be clear and consistent when making corrections

If nurses need to correct a notation on a chart, they should draw a line through improper or incorrect charting and place the word "error" immediately after the entry and have a nurse manager sign next to it. Whiteout should never be used on a chart.

Only used approved abbreviations/shorthand

Nurses should never use shorthand or abbreviations that are not widely used in the medical community and are not easy to understand. One of the JCAHO's seven National Patient Safety Goals (NPSG) requires hospitals to standardize the ways in which staff abbreviate or symbolize expressions throughout the organization, including developing a list of confusing abbreviations, acronyms, and symbols that staff should not use. To this end, the JCAHO has developed a minimum list of dangerous abbreviations, acronyms, and symbols in time for you to comply with the 2004 NPSG that went into effect January 1, 2004.

Note medication times

Because of the increased efforts federal regulators have focused on preventing medication errors, it's critical for nurses to accurately chart any and all medication situations with patients. Good medication documentation must include the time the nurse gave a medication, the administration route, and the patient's response. Continued monitoring of a patient's reaction to medications is important, as well.

Record "unusual" incidents

Nurses should always chart all of their observations, their actions, and the patient's response to medications and treatment. List any "unusual" incidents, such as the patient becoming aggressive or combative, and subsequent safety precautions taken to protect the patient. Patients perceived as "difficult" may be acting differently because of the introduction of a new medication or a drug interaction.

Include conversations with physicians

Nurses should also note any conversations they had with a physician to discuss a patient's behavior, order tests, or request medications. They should also ensure that they date and time each chart entry and follow each entry they make with their signature.

Avoid generalizations

Nurses' documentation should be clear, concise, and specific. There should be no generalizations. Instead of saying "patient seems to be improving," a nurse needs to describe the patient's progress. Avoid using labels such as "noncompliant", "combative", or "difficult" to describe patients. Instead, note their behavior, for instance, "patient refused to eat dinner or take meds" or "patient struggled with nurse assistant who attempted to help feed him his meals."

Complete comprehensive follow-ups to falls/injuries

If a patient sustains a fall or injury, nurses must list how the patient was injured, and steps that are being taken to ensure the patient doesn't sustain further injuries.

Record discharge education

When a patient is discharged, it's imperative for nurses to note all education and discharge instructions given to the family. This is especially critical in cases of difficult family members who have expressed dissatisfaction regarding the patient's care and may decide to file a lawsuit.

Never sign a colleague's chart

Nurses should never make or sign a chart entry for a colleague. In turn, nurses should never ask a colleague to make a chart entry for one of their own patients. Nurses need to be reminded that their signature on a chart makes them as responsible for the entry as the original recorder.

Accurate documentation provides nurses with a consistent approach in dealing with difficult patients. If a patient was combative the last time he or she was hospitalized, an accurate record might illustrate to staff what methods proved effective in subduing the patient.

For staff to use patient charts for this purpose, they must use the guidance above and consistently create patient charts that include vital information and are legible, well-organized, and easy to use.

Working with the noncompliant patient

Noncompliant patients are patients who do not follow prescribed treatment plans and repeatedly miss appointments. These patients are often candidates for becoming difficult, and they pose a serious threat for litigation.

Acts of noncompliance, however, are not always deliberate on the part of the patient. Often when patients are noncompliant, it is simply that they did not understand discharge instructions or do not feel comfortable asking questions.

This emphasizes some of the challenges we identified with difficult patient populations in Chapter 1.

A noncompliant patient may be a senior citizen who does not understand a new technology, a non-English-speaking immigrant confused by a translation, or an uninsured patient worried about how her or she will afford the treatment plan or appointment.

Keep detailed chart notes of all of your conversations with noncompliant patients. If a patient refuses treatment, his or her medical record must contain a description of the examination, treatment, or both, if applicable, that was refused by the patient. It's critical for nurses to also clearly document that further tests and/or treatments were offered by the facility before the patient refused. If the patient declines to have further treatment, the hospital must show in writing the risks/benefits of the treatment refused.

In addition, the hospital must take all reasonable steps to secure the individual's written informed refusal (or that of a person acting on his or her behalf). A hospital cannot be left without recourse if an individual refused treatment, refused to sign a statement to that effect, and leaves against medical advice. Nurses should document those facts.

Documenting the violent patient

In the event that patients become combative, nursing staff should complete a workplace violence form to document the incident.

Additionally, nursing staff should document, in the nurse's notes, a factual and objective narrative of what occurred. As a Medicare Condition of Participation, hospitals are required to provide workplace violence training that is proportionate to an employee's level of risk. In other words, the employees at greatest risk, such as ED or psych nurses, would have the highest level of training.

Documenting episodes of violence can help nursing managers determine which staff members may require additional training as well as areas in the unit that may need additional safety measures.

Documenting a violent patient is also helpful when a patient is frequently admitted to a facility. The documentation can provide staff with a clear picture of what triggered the patient to become combative in the past, as well as alert staff that the patient is prone to violent behavior.

Working to improve your documentation system

Consider putting together a hospital task force to develop a smoother system for managing patient information and reducing the amount of staff documentation.

By streamlining forms, your task force can create a controlled, consistent method of documentation across departments. This improved documentation system can help nurses by eliminating repetitive documentation and freeing up more time for patient care.

Your team's goal should be to determine how to make it easier for nurses and physicians to locate patient information and improve communication of this information between departments.

Discuss how to document pertinent information, eliminate duplicate charting, and streamline the documentation process. Brainstorm ways to simplify the process, minimize the amount of time nurses spend on documentation, and create a better flow throughout the hospitals. How does your hospital currently document and assess difficult patients or situations? If you don't already have protocols in place, this is the time to consider how you want to address these situations. Your efforts can also lead to improved patient satisfaction.

If you do develop new forms, be sure to introduce new documents with a well-organized and consistent in-service for staff.

Involving your risk management department

When nurses are faced with difficult patient situations, it's imperative that you instruct them to involve your hospital's risk management department immediately.

The role of your organization's risk management department is to present, identify, evaluate, and minimize exposure to liability. Its role becomes much more difficult if it is not made aware of a difficult patient situation promptly.

Risk Managers can work with nursing staff on problems such as:

- Unexpected complications relating to a procedure or equipment
- Poor treatment outcomes
- Angry patients or families
- Letters or calls from attorneys
- Communications from a state board

Remember that patients and their families have the right to sue regardless whether negligence has occurred. By involving your risk management department quickly, they can work with nursing staff to clear up misunderstandings and avoid lawsuits and further hostile interactions.

Understanding informed consent

Informed consent describes the process whereby a fully informed patient participates in choices about his or her health care. Every patient has the legal and ethical rights to determine what happens to his or her body. The informed consent process should be seen as an invitation to the patient to participate in his or her health care decisions.

Informed consent gives all patients the opportunity to be informed participants in their health care decisions. Complete informed consents include a discussion of the following:

- The nature of the decision/procedure
- Reasonable alternatives to the proposed intervention
- The relevant risks, benefits, and uncertainties related to each alternative
- Assessment of patient comprehension
- Acceptance of the intervention by the patient

Informed consent is not just a signature on a piece of paper. Rather, it is a process by which the individual performing the procedure provides information to the patient. The form is simply verification that the process occurred. It is incumbent on the person performing the procedure to obtain informed consent and document it accordingly.

In order for the patient's consent to be valid, he or she must be considered competent to make the decision and the consent must be voluntary. Nurses need to clearly explain that patients are participating in a decision, not simply signing a form.

Competence is the ability to

- express a choice
- understand information relevant to making a treatment decision
- appreciate the significance of that information for one's own situation, especially concerning one's illness and the probable consequences of one's treatment options
- reason with relevant information so as to engage in a logical process of weighing treatment options.

The absence of any of these brings into question the individual's ability to provide informed consent.

If a nurse is not sure as to whether a patient is competent to make his or her own decisions, the nurse should first assess the patient's ability to

- understand his or her medical condition
- understand the risks associated with the options being presented
- communicate a decision based on that understanding

A crucial aspect of the nurse's patient advocacy role is the obligation to ensure that medical interventions are not undertaken unless the patient fully comprehends the details. If this does not occur, nurses should notify the physician that informed consent has not been given and that the patient requires additional information.

If a patient is found incompetent or unable to make health care decisions, a surrogate decision maker must be appointed.

Proper informed consent and its medical record documentation includes:

1. Diagnosis of the problem
2. Nature of the recommended treatment and benefit
3. Risks, discomforts, disability, or disfiguring aspects of proposed medical treatments or surgical procedures
4. Realistic expectation of outcome
5. Realistic expectation of outcome or risks if the condition is not treated
6. Alternative treatments, including additional consultation
7. Identity of the treating physician and/or surgeon

Although not every treatment requires a patient's informed consent, professional ethics suggest that physicians and nursing staff provide it routinely. Discussion of informed consent must be documented if the treatment could cause serious side effects.

Revocation of informed consent

Patients have the right to revoke informed consent at any time, either verbally or in writing. This is more common than it used to be, and it evolves from the noncompliant patient who will not accept the recommendations made to him or her.

If this happens, nurses should notify the patient's primary physician immediately, and the revocation should be immediately noted in the patient's chart. The patient should be required to fill out a form that describes the recommended treatment, the reason the treatment is needed, and the consequences of not having the treatment. The patient should be required to sign this form, acknowledging that everyone involved understands who is making the decision and who is responsible.

If a patient revokes consent out of fear and/or misunderstanding, it may be appropriate to offer additional counsel. It is never appropriate to use coercion.

Documenting phone calls from patients and families

When a patient or family member calls your nursing unit with a concern or your advice nurse with after-hours questions, it's important to document the phone call in the patient's chart.

Failure to properly document these conversations could come back to hurt you in court. Often these conversations include an exchange of clinical information that is not documented clearly in the patient's chart—if it is documented at all.

Consider developing a notepad with preprinted areas for recording phone conversations with patients or family members. Be sure the pad has enough space for nurses to include all the important details. It should include the following:

1. Time and date the call was received
2. Name of person who called
3. Name of person who received the call
4. If and when the call was returned to the patient
5. Issues/treatments that were discussed
6. Condition or clinical status of the patient
7. Physician's name
8. Physician's response to the question/concern

Without documentation, in the event of litigation, it becomes very hard for nurses to defend details of discussions and recall specific instructions.

Clear documentation reduces liability and can be an indispensable performance improvement tool for your staff and your organization.

Chapter 10

LEADING YOUR STAFF TOWARD IMPROVED SERVICE AND SATISFACTION

CHAPTER 10

Leading Your Staff Toward Improved Service and Satisfaction

Every medical facility should have a customer service program in place. Customer satisfaction should be a daily part of everyone's job, not just a topic to be addressed when you receive a patient complaint.

Does your facility have a strong customer service program in place? Are nurses aware of your facility's policy? Are patients routinely surveyed to determine their satisfaction with their treatment outcome and your facility's environment?

Getting patient input is important, as is constructively sharing the results of patients surveys so that quality of care can be improved. All too often, staff hear only negative comments. If a patient verbally praises a member of your staff, ask him or her to put those comments into writing (even offer to provide a pen and paper!). Consider posting positive feedback in staff rooms or sharing positive feedback during report. Everyone likes to receive positive reinforcement.

Has your staff ever undergone formal customer service training? Although many nurses might claim customer service training is nothing more than common sense, offering training at your facility for all staff can reap the rewards of patient satisfaction. Facilities that have implemented strong customer service training programs report a decrease in complaints and an increase in compliments. Many educators use successful customer services programs by multinational corporations such as Disney, Starbucks, and Nordstrom as models that keep both customers and employees happy.

The importance of nurse leader rounding

Nurse rounding is one of the best ways for nurse leaders to identify potential difficult patients early on in their stay. As we have discussed throughout this book, early identification and appropriate communication are crucial to managing difficult patients. Also, rounding is a vehicle for managers and other administrators to win the respect of their staff and lead the entire department toward improved customer service and patient satisfaction.

Quint Studer, CEO of the Studer Group, a consulting firm that helps guide organizations through major changes, brings his 20 years of experience in health care to thousands of hospitals each year, through his workshops and materials on creating organizational excellence.

Studer has identified nurse manager rounding as one of the most important tools for improving employee and patient satisfaction.

When nurse managers make the rounds, their goals are to:
- fix and monitor systems
- ensure goals were accomplished
- model desired behavior
- talk to individuals in the department and update information

Managers should have a key question to ask staff such as, "Do you have what you need to do your job today?" If the staff need something, it's an opportunity to figure out why they don't have it, without blaming administration.

Managers should also reward and recognize staff during rounding. You should ask questions or make observations to assess staff are performing in the manner you are trying to achieve and then specifically recognize staff who exhibit the desired behavior. The key is recognizing and rewarding behavior that gets repeated.

Studer recommends that nurse managers and other administrators set aside time each day for rounding—for example, you may want to begin meetings after 10 a.m., with the understanding that the time before 10 a.m. is spent rounding in work areas.

Nurse leader rounding is done to fix systems; ensure that staff have tools and equipment in place; identify, decrease, and remove barriers; and reward and recognize staff.

Nurse rounding and patient satisfaction

Studer's research also shows that nurse manager rounding has a profound impact on patient satisfaction. He lists the following as keys to ensuring that your rounding will have a positive effect on patient satisfaction:

1. Set expectations. When a nurse manager rounds, it is important that he or she set expectations for patients. The nurse leader introduces herself to the patient and then lets the patient and family (if available) know that the goal of the hospital is to provide excellent care. Use the same language as in the hospital's survey tool. After welcoming the patient say, "Our goal is to provide you with very good care. If at any time you do not feel you are receiving very good care, please let your nurse or me know."

2. Use key words at key times. If the patient's nurse has written her name on a white board in the room, use key words to reinforce this: "Oh, I see that Stacey is your nurse today. If you have any positive comments about Stacey, please write them on your patient satisfaction survey." Then say, "Do you know what your schedule is today?" This is a way to reinforce to the patient his or her role in the care being provided. Fostering this understanding with your patients during rounding should improve your patient satisfaction scores.

3. Use closing statements. No patient contact is complete without a closing statement. Studer noted that the best physicians always end a patient encounter with a closing statement that can be phrased as a question, for example, "Before I leave, do you have any other questions?" This brings the visit to a close, further defines the role of the patient and his or her family, and may reduce follow-up phone calls to the hospital for more information later on.

Protecting yourself and your staff from lawsuits

Occasionally, situations with difficult patients will escalate to the point of litigation. To protect you and your staff from claims of malpractice, ensure that you are familiar with and your staff adhere to the following advice:

Know the law

Your state's Nurse Practice Act is the standard by which a nurse's professional behavior will be judged in any potential malpractice case. If it can be conclusively shown that a nurse acted in accordance with the law, the case will likely be dismissed before it goes to trial.

Keep education current

Lawyers are less likely to name nurses in a lawsuit who keeps up with their continuing education requirements than those nurses who have let their training slip.

Encourage nurses to act as patient advocates.

If a doctor fails to act in the face of compelling patient distress, encourage nurses to always bring the case to their nurse manager. Empower nurses to act as advocates for their patients and look out for their best interests. Inform them that there will be no adverse consequences for questioning a physician's authority, but that staying silent could ultimately cost them their nursing license.

Review your policies and procedures

Stay up to date with your organization's policies and procedures. What are your policies concerning patients rights and responsibilities, how staff respond to angry or grieving families, and so on. Have your new hires and contract nursing staff been sufficiently informed?

Document everything

Having a written record to prove that you and your staff acted in accordance with the accepted standards of practice is crucial. As discussed in Chapter 9, good charting is a primary defense against liability in a malpractice suit. Train nursing staff to include all of their assessments in the documentation as well as evaluations of how treatments or interventions worked, patient noncompliance, communication with physicians on any of these issues, and signs of patient distress. Teach staff to never document care before its delivered or add to the record after a significant amount of time has passed. Also, nurses should know never to alter records after the fact.

Retain a sense of composure and compassion

It is often hard to act kind or compassionate to someone who is angry or acting difficult, but studies show that if a patient likes his or her nurse he or she is less likely to sue that nurse. Teach nursing staff, that if a patient complains about something they've done, it's more effective to correct the problem without becoming defensive.

Simplify patient education

An important factor in reducing liability risk is patient education. Having nurses work with patients to teach them about their condition, treatment plan, coverage for follow-up procedures, and other similar topics increases the likelihood that the patient will follow instructions and not become noncompliant. Noncompliant patients are often the same patients who seek attorneys when care falls short of their expectations.

Five things patients never want to hear from your nurses

As we have discussed throughout this book, good communication is the key to patient and staff satisfaction, so it is important to recognize instances when what your nurse says negatively affects patient satisfaction.

In her motivational seminars to health care professionals, Susan Keane Baker lists five statements patients never want to hear. Are you or your nursing staff guilty of uttering any of the following phrases?

1. "I have no idea."

Comment: It's virtually impossible to say this with enough compassion in your voice to overcome the patient's perception what you really mean is, "I'm glad that I don't know, and therefore unable to help you. I don't want to know, and I don't care."

2. "We're short-staffed."

Comment: When patients hear this, they may think, "Poor dear, she's doing her best," or they may think, "Gosh, I'd better not let her go, or I may never see her again." If your nurses prefer clinging, anxious patients, comments about staffing can help guarantee that they will have plenty.

3. "I hate to speak ill of a co-worker, but between you and me…"

Comment: Expressions of critical peer review made to patients decreases their trust and confidence in the entire organization. Patients also will worry that their nurse is criticizing them to others.

4. "You're not our only patient, you know."

Comment: Patients translate this as, "You're not important to us." Consider instead, "Is there anything I can do for you before I go to answer the call bell for another patient?"

5. "There's nothing we can do about it."

Comment: This statement conveys that a nurse is powerless or, worse yet, incompetent, especially if other people or organizations *can* do something about a similar request or situation.

Bringing out the best in your nurses

Recognize nurses who effectively handle difficult patients and difficult situations. Encourage them to share their strategies at staff meetings.

Acknowledge that nursing can often be a challenging profession, and look for opportunities throughout the year to celebrate your successes and renew your staff's commitment to choosing a profession as lifelong caregivers.

To promote unity among your staff, try this technique used by some nurse managers: Give staff members pens and paper at a staff meeting and ask them to take a few minutes to write out their positive comments (anonymously or not) about one another. Have them submit all comments to the leader of the meeting, who then separates them into piles for each employee. He or she then reads the comments aloud to the group. This promotes a positive outlook among staff members and increases employees' feelings of self-worth. Be sure to pass the papers on to the employee who is being complimented.

Helping your organization become a leader in employee satisfaction

Try to help your hospital move toward becoming a leader in employee satisfaction. Nurse managers cannot change an entire corporate culture, but you and your colleagues can implement programs that ensure a better working environment for nurses. These programs will not only help with employee satisfaction, they will also help you retain nursing staff.

Many hospitals have already recognized and embraced the link between employee satisfaction and patient satisfaction. Baptist Healthcare Corp., of Pensacola, FL, has been recognized as a leader in this area. That organization's culture is characterized by:

- A "no secrets, open book" environment in which staff members are "in the know" about customer and employee satisfaction and financial results through a number of information-sharing venues such as employee forums and reports that are distributed throughout the organization
- Reward and recognition programs to acknowledge and empower employees
- Leadership teams accountable not only for their department's financial results, but also for employee satisfaction rates

For the past two years, *Fortune* magazine has named Baptist Healthcare as one of the "Top 100 Best Places to Work in America."

Other hospitals have implemented programs promoting staff learning and development, and an open culture in which nursing staff are invited to voice their opinions and do not fear retribution.

Empowering your nursing staff to bring about change

Consider asking nursing staff to fill out surveys after three- and six-month periods of employment. Continue to do this on a six-month basis to assess staffers' experiences in the organization. Part of the survey can ask nurses anonymously for ways to improve the patient-care process in their unit, as well as determine areas of improvement.

Some facilities hold twice-yearly breakfasts or dinners at which nursing staff can meet with the senior vice president of nursing and other nurse administrators to share their concerns and suggestions.

Establish a nonpunitive reporting system to encourage nurses to report errors. To accomplish this, many facilities are urging nurses and other clinical staff to admit error, even in the absence of legal action. Some hospitals are offering staff rewards, such as gift certificates, to encourage reporting of errors and to motivate staff to come up with solutions.

Many facilities have found that the key to increasing job satisfaction among nurses is to use fewer outside nurses, and to emphasize education and promotional opportunities, as well as giving nurses more authority. Nurse managers can work to help make all nurses a key part of the hospital's governance process. Consider developing a council of nurses that meets regularly to discuss patient care and administrative issues. Also see if it's possible within your facility to have nurses sit on interdisciplinary councils, where they can express their concerns to physicians and others.

Tight-budget training strategies for nurse managers

Looking to offer staff development programs for nurses, but don't have a hefty budget?

Consider in-house resources

Would your Employee Assistance Program offer a complimentary workshop on reducing stress? Can you barter services with your physical therapy department for mini neck and shoulder massages to be offered twice a month to nursing staff?

Look to the community for workshop ideas and speakers

Take a poll among nurses to learn which topics they would like additional training. Geriatric care is a popular and pertinent topic with the aging Baby Boomers, yet many nursing schools are cutting programs that teach nurses how to deal with patients who suffer from severe cognitive impairment. Invite your local Alzheimer's Association chapter to conduct a workshop for nurses on how to recognize signs of dementia and how to effectively care for the growing number of Alzheimer's and dementia patients.

Ask your human resources department to check with your local four-year college or university about the possibility of offering bachelor of science in nursing programs onsite, making it more convenient for nursing staff to take courses.

Invite a local law enforcement agency to discuss violence prevention or arrange for the health department to conduct a workshop on how nurses can reduce their risk of contracting Hepatitis C through inadvertent needle sticks and other mishaps.

Embracing new technology

Technology can help nurses work smarter, not harder. Has your facility invested in technology? Often nurse managers can serve as catalysts for technology in the workplace. If you hear of a technological innovation that you think will help your staff do their jobs better, present your ideas to administrators.

One of the areas in which new technology can help nurses most is documentation. Research has shown that nurses spend as much as 30% of their time doing paperwork—much of which occurs at the shift's end and beyond, forcing many nurses to work overtime. Think how nurses could be using this precious time caring for patients instead!

New bedside documentation allows nurses to chart in real-time as they care for patients, which also reduces the chance for errors.

Some facilities have also started equipping nurses with four-channel portable telephones that allow them to stay at the patient's bedside and still be instantly in touch with other nursing staff, physicians, and departments, such as pharmacy and labs.

Chapter 11

ASSESSING YOUR STAFF'S SKILLS IN DEALING WITH DIFFICULT PATIENTS AND FAMILIES

CHAPTER 11

Assessing Your Staff's Skills in Dealing with Difficult Patients and Families

Now that you've transformed your nursing staff into experts in patient satisfaction, how will you rate them on their strategies for handling difficult patient situations?

If your organization does not currently rate nurses on patient satisfaction, consider working with your human resources department to add a category on your performance appraisal that measures a nurse's competency in this area. Define performance objectives and state the desired outcomes.

As a nurse manager, empower yourself to go beyond your hospital's standard appraisal form if it's inadequate in reviewing how nurses handle difficult patients. Focus on the nurse's competency in this area even if the form doesn't require it.

Is "handling difficult patients" a competency?

A competency is the demonstration of one or more skills based on knowledge derived from educational programs or experience.

Observing and measuring competencies for every staff member assures hospital leaders that the people delivering care at their facility are doing so safely and efficiently.

Establishing and implementing an effective program for verifying and validating the skills and abilities of staff is the key to complying with the Joint Commission on Accreditation of Healthcare Organizations (JCAHO's) competency-related standards, which are found in the human resources function. A well-developed competency assessment program will bring value to the patient, the employee, and the organization.

Out of the thousands of competencies that must be performed every day by employees, the organization must decide which need to be assessed, the frequency with which they will be assessed, and the manner in which they will be assessed. A logical starting point for making this decision is your department's job descriptions.

Competency-based job descriptions

The job description for each of your staff members should be based on his or her duties and responsibilities. A competency-based job description would state these duties and responsibilities in terms of practice standards, or the way in which they are to be demonstrated.

Although the skills we have discussed in this book have become requirements for most organizations, there is very little mention of the skills and responsibilities required for handling difficult patients or families in most job descriptions. There are usually references to skills such as problem solving, communicating appropriately, and dispute resolution, but usually these expectations are not clearly spelled out.

An example of this can be found in the following excerpt from a sample job description for a staff nurse. These job responsibilities appeared under the heading "Interpersonal skills."

    A. *Demonstrates flexibility, as well as attitude and actions that are conducive to effective working relationships.*

    B. *Effectively communicates information to others.*

    C. *Deals with conflict situations within the unit and when interfacing with other departments/groups.*

    D. *Communicates and interacts with clients, families, and external representatives. Recognizes the effects of stress on patients and their families and initiates actions that facilitate coping."*

Competency-based job descriptions should couple the skills and responsibilities associated with handling difficult patient or family situations, including, for example, cultural competencies and de-escalation techniques with how these skills must be demonstrated.

For example, perhaps your department requires staff to attend an annual education program on handling difficult patients and the related federal and state regulations. The staff member's responsibility is to attend the mandatory annual education program. However, a competency-based job description would state that the employee "identifies potentially difficult patients and uses de-escalation techniques to prevent confrontations." This statement combines the responsibility and the expected practice standards used to assess the competency by stating that the employee can demonstrate what he or she learned in the annual program.

Ongoing competency validation

Organizations validate competencies not only to comply with JCAHO requirements, but also to ensure that their employees are performing the skills and responsibilities appropriate to their job descriptions. Often, organizations have a process for assessing competencies before the employee is hired and at the end of the orientation period, but there must be an assurance that this is an ongoing effort.

During any given year, organizations add new technologies, new treatment plans, and new procedures. You may decide that the competencies related to handling difficult patients and families need to be assessed annually. When and how do you do this?

The formal review of competency usually occurs as part of the employee's annual performance review. Keep in mind, however, that this is more than just a review of the employee's ability to meet the contractual expectations of the job for which he or she was hired. This is an evaluation of the employee's continued ability to perform his or her job. As a result, many organizations designate a separate "Skills Day" for assessing competencies.

Some of the most effective methods for assessing interpersonal competencies related to handling difficult patients include the following:

- Demonstration/observation
- Case study/discussion group
- Peer review
- Self-assessment
- Presentation
- Simulation/drill

Evaluating customer service standards

When developing the competencies for your department, involve front-line nurses in setting the standards. Ask nurses the top 10 things they want patients to remember for them and have staff commit to upholding the goals and standards developed by their peers.

At the time of their yearly performance reviews, nurses should be evaluated on how they have incorporated these service standards into their daily routines. Nurse managers should then evaluate and reward nurses based at least in part on their success at delivering good service.

When interviewing potential new employees, nursing managers should discuss customer service principles as they apply to the organization's mission statement and service standards. Ask new hires how they exemplify these standards based on their past work experience and ask which techniques nurses have used in the past to handle difficult patients.

Performance reviews

Although many nursing managers dread the task of conducting performance reviews, when done well, they can boost morale and enhance productivity among nursing staff. Given a nurse manager's hectic schedule, performance reviews also allow for designated times to meet with staff and have an open conversation about job duties, expectations, problems, and concerns.

Recording anecdotal notes about your observation of staff's experiences with difficult patients and families—and maintaining them all year—is a good method for ensuring that the review covers the entire year. Anecdotal notes should be maintained by the manager and reflect not only opportunities for improvement but also positive aspects of performance.

These review sessions provide an opportunity for you to annually assess each staff member's performance in this area, praising good techniques and offering performance improvement strategies.

When conducting a performance review, nurse managers should have employees fill out a detailed self-evaluation form, describing their strengths, weaknesses, and accomplishments. Discuss ways in which nurses can improve their handling of specific difficult patient situations. The form should include questions such as the following:

- Do you need additional training?
- Do you lack essential tools or support?
- In which areas would you like to receive additional training?

Use this data to decide on areas of growth for the coming year. Remember that performance reviews should never be a complete surprise to nurses, and they aren't a replacement for giving nursing staff input on a regular basis. Plan to give nurses specific feedback on their jobs at least once a week. If you catch them in the act of handling a patient situation well, compliment them on the spot.

Some hospitals have incorporated interpersonal skills such as respect, courtesy, listening, and anticipating patients' needs as part of employees' annual performance appraisal. Appraisals are conducted after employees are offered skill-building workshops on topics such as how best to keep a patient's family informed of their loved ones' condition. Nurse managers can assist by being good role models, coaching nursing staff on best practices, and encouraging nurses to avoid medical jargon when talking with patients and their families.

Some guidance for evaluating customer service skills during performance reviews is as follows:

- Avoid using general behaviors as criteria in annual performance reviews such as, "pleasant demeanor." Address specific skills instead, such as "Answers phones in the unit promptly and always responds to inquiries from patient families in a timely and polite manner."

- Report critical incidents that take place throughout the year. It's often hard for nurse managers to sit down and recall the specifics of a nurse's job performance over the past year. Many nursing managers have found it useful to compile anecdotal notes of critical incidents on an ongoing basis. These are reports of an employee's behavior that are out of the ordinary, either positive or negative.

- Consider using a 360-degree evaluation. Many hospitals have begun utilizing this method, which combines elements of peer review, to produce a more comprehensive array of feedback generated from as many perspectives as possible. In this model, physicians evaluate nurses, nurses evaluate physicians, nursing assistants evaluate nurses, and your nursing staff evaluates you. A 360-degree evaluation uncovers workplace behavior and patterns that might otherwise go unnoticed through other top-down evaluation methods. Feedback on a 360-degree evaluation comes from the people a nurse interacts with on a daily basis. They have a working knowledge of how a nurse handles difficult patient situations and can provide valuable feedback on situations that might not be observed by nurse managers.

Monitoring staff satisfaction

Even hospitals with the best intentions can fail at implementing patient satisfaction programs, if they neglect to address the needs of their internal customers.

When you first introduce a new program for handling difficult patients and increasing patient satisfaction, you will probably be met with resistance from some of your more skeptical staff members.

Nurses will probably wonder how they can possibly find the time to attend meetings or training sessions. As a nurse manager, it's imperative that you address these concerns, and also set the tone for changes in your unit. You will need to assure your nursing staff that your medical center's management is committed to exploring new ways of dealing with difficult patient situations, and that the solutions will benefit both nursing staff and patients. Ensure that you provide coverage so that nurses can participate on teams and be paid for their time. As a follow-up measure, be sure to share results and actions taken and to celebrate successes at staff meetings. You can also post results and best practices on a bulletin board in the staff room.

An effective nurse manager needs to put as much effort into keeping nurses happy as they put into keeping patients happy. They realize the importance of regularly offering support to their nursing staff and practicing active listening.

When a nurse comes to you with a complaint about a difficult patient situation, don't dismiss him or her by saying that you are "reviewing the situation" and will "address the problem." Say, specifically, how you plan to address the concerns and describe the actions you plan to take. Involve nurses in resolving the problem and empower them to be part of the solution. Thank your staff member for bringing the problem to your attention and assure him or her you will act on their concerns. Ignoring a staff member's request breeds resentment and communicates to staff that you don't care about them or their working conditions.

Many nurses are critical of patient satisfaction programs or new methods of patient care because they feel administrators are asking them to take on additional responsibilities when they are already overworked. How can tired and stressed nurses be expected to offer world-class customer service?

When implementing a patient satisfaction program, nurse managers need to review their expectations with nurses. Let staff know you are working to make their jobs easier, not harder. If you are implementing programs such as passing out snacks to patient families who are waiting in the ED, secure a volunteer to do this task and inform nurses that you don't expect them to take on the added responsibility.

Also involve nurses in structuring employee recognition programs. Use their input and involve them in programs where peers can recognize other nurses for their expertise in handling particularly difficult patient situations.

Recognize nurses who handle difficult patients with finesse and ask them to share their techniques at the next unit staff meeting.

It is essential that you, as a nurse manager, go beyond simply educating staff on strategies for dealing with difficult patients. You should consider developing a process that fits best with your organization. This might mean developing a new process for competency assessment or reworking your current one.

You also have a responsibility to monitor your staff's satisfaction, motivate them to be better, and reward them for their contributions. Future success in the early identification and effective management of difficult patients depends on your ability to carry through on these responsibilities.

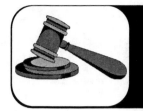

CASE STUDY: A CONNECTICUT HOSPITAL'S PROGRAM CAN SERVE AS MODEL FOR REWARDING STAFF FOR BEST PRACTICES

What makes a hospital a great place for nurses to work? How do you support your nursing staff while also keeping patients and their families happy? Griffin Hospital, in Derby, CT, has been recognized for three consecutive years by Fortune Magazine as one of the "100 Best Companies to Work For in America." The culture at Griffin is defined by increased employee satisfaction and retention and generally high morale among staff.

Employees are recognized for exemplary service year-round, not just during performance reviews, and are given the tools and training needed to succeed in their jobs. Below are some of Griffin's unique employee programs.

Orientation

Each employee of Griffin Hospital is required to attend a mandatory two-day orientation program prior to beginning work-related duties at the hospital. In addition to learning the Griffin patient-centered philosophy as told by the chief executive officer (CEO) and vice-president, new employees receive a summary of information on topics such as human resources, safety, standard precautions, legal issues, and a brief tour of the hospital.

TIP: An employee orientation can provide a good first step in giving new hires an overview of how your facility expects them to handle difficult patients and how to document these situations.

Recognition programs

ITIP—Griffin employees are recognized monthly through the "I Take It Personally" Program, or "ITIP." The employee population is broken down into four divisions: nursing, service, support, and ancillary. One employee from each division is named Employee of the Month.

A themed celebration to recognize these four employees takes place each month in the cafeteria hosted by the CEO with the help of the reigning Employee of the Year.   The program is designed to publicly recognize and reward employee behavior, which improves patient/client satisfaction.

CASE STUDY: A CONNECTICUT HOSPITAL'S PROGRAM CAN SERVE AS MODEL FOR REWARDING STAFF FOR BEST PRACTICES, CONT.

Employee winners receive a bonus check for this distinction. A companion program is the Department of the Quarter program, which is designed to single out departments that excel in meeting quarterly or annual objectives or go the extra mile in assisting patients, guests, or fellow employees. The Annual Employee Service Awards are held each May to honor those employees with five or more years of service, each monthly ITIP winner, and all four Department of the Quarter honorees.

The highlight of the evening is the selection of the Employee of the Year and Department of the Year.

TIP: Consider a special category for nurse innovations. If one of your nurses has come up with a creative way of dealing with difficult patients, be sure to recognize this practice.

Never Fear, Never Quit—Recognizing that dealing with difficult patients or families represents just one piece of health care that can often be stressful, employees at Griffin are encouraged to attend monthly motivational "Never Fear Never Quit" programs. These programs include lectures on integrity, perseverance, and authentication, and create a forum for employees to voice their concerns and opinions. A number of employees are selected to become "Spark Plugs" and take a leadership role in increasing employee morale and encouraging positive behavior from co-workers.

TIP: Think about what you do to motivate employees on a regular basis. You can often invite members of the community to give a motivational lecture at no cost. Consider a speaker on stress management or dealing with difficult people. Check with your local college or Chamber of Commerce for speakers with excellent credentials.

Spot Recognition Program—Employees are also recognized "on the spot" with the "Spot Recognition Program." This program recognized employees who go above and beyond their duties with small tokens of appreciation such as movie passes, gift certificates, discounted coupons, free coffee and donuts, or just a card to say thanks. Managers and directors are encouraged to pull these items from "Tool Boxes" given to them by administration.